TRAINING PLANS FOR EVERY CYCLING LEVEL

CYCLING WORKOUT HANDBOOK

IMPROVE FITNESS WITH 100 OF THE BEST CYCLING WORKOUTS

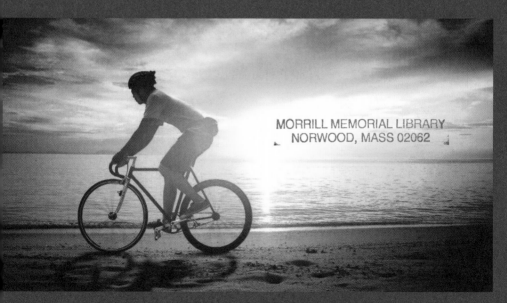

TERRI SCHNEIDER

getfitnow

Your health starts here! Workouts, nutrition, motivation, community…everything you need to build a better body from the inside out!

Visit us at www.getfitnow.com for videos, workouts, nutrition, recipes, community tips, and more!

Cycling Workout Handbook

Text Copyright © 2018 Terri Schneider

Library of Congress Cataloging-in-Publication. Data is available.

ISBN: 978-1-57826-770-5

BOOK DESIGN BY CAROLYN KASPER

Printed in the United States

10 9 8 7 6 5 4 3 2 1

CONTENTS

CYCLING WORKOUTS 43

About the Author 215

BENEFITS OF FITNESS CYCLING

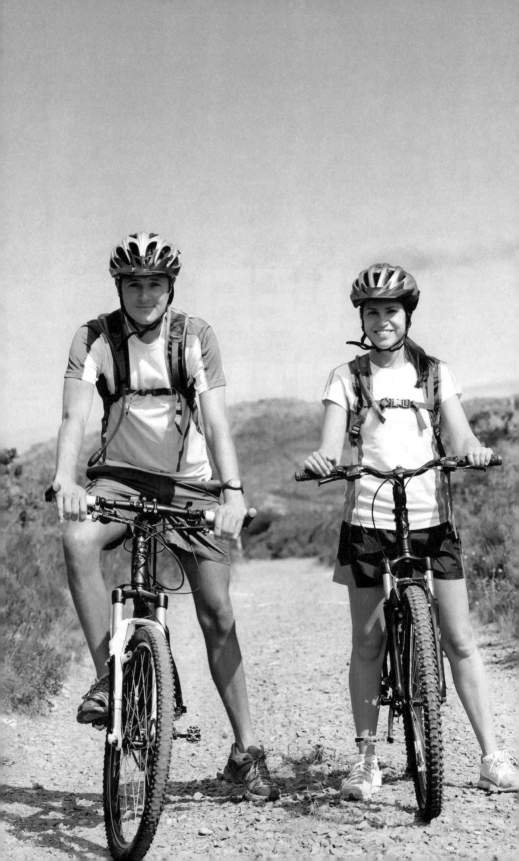

Are you just getting into cycling? Are you interested in adding cycling to your fitness program, looking to increase your overall fitness level, or just want to take on a longer ride than you've done prior?

If so, the programs and organized workout sessions in *Cycling Workout Handbook* are for *you*.

My cycling life began at a young age when I started riding for fun and transportation. This continued on into college and, alongside my normal run training, let me easily transition a daily activity into triathlons. Throughout my triathlon training, I enjoyed increasing my pedaling distance, always looking for the next beautiful place to ride even further.

Trading in my road bike, I gravitated toward mountain biking, which in turn led me to adventure racing and various bike adventures around the world, which continue today. All the while, I've continued to ride for fun and transportation. Being in consistent cycling shape continues to open doors to a variety of new experiences, all from the seat of my bike. Believe me when I say that the possibilities open to you when you jump on your bike are endless!

Adventure isn't cycling's only benefit; not only does it get us out exploring the roads and trails, it extends our cardiovascular fitness and bolsters our total lower body strength—all in a non-weight bearing mode. An organized and well-crafted week of cycling training offers you wellness benefits beyond your wildest dreams while still keeping fun and exploration at the forefront of your fitness.

Studies have shown that even a minimal amount of endurance training per week will reduce tendencies toward anxiety, stress, and depression, while improving one's quality of sleep and overall mood and mental focus. These benefits are best realized through achieving diversity in intensity, recovery, and distance within each session and within each week. This diversity of training (inclusive of recovery days) promotes the three aspects that trigger our body to grow stronger, faster, and more proficient.

Another important element is consistency. When training over many weeks, it's important to stick to your plan and stay consistent. I've incorporated all these training elements into a cycling-specific program, presented here as the *Cycling Workout Handbook*, to offer everyone a chance to participate in this motivating and highly productive process.

So again: if you have been looking to make cycling a part of a diverse cross-training fitness program, this handbook is for you. And if your goal is to ride longer and stronger than you ever have, *Cycling Workout Handbook* will get you there!

CYCLING BASICS

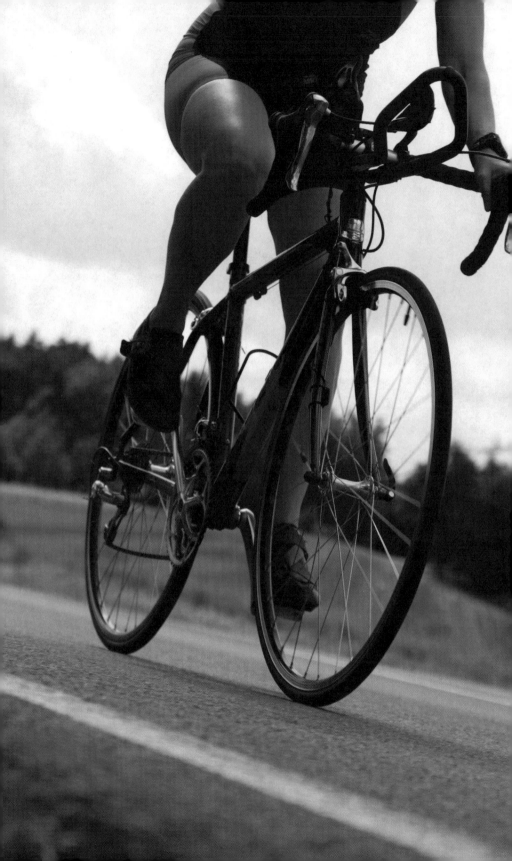

Acquiring a Bike

When looking for your perfect bike, there are several pieces to the puzzle, including how much you're looking to spend, what you'll use the bike for, frame material and geometry, and where to purchase your bike. Gathering these pieces takes some effort but is well worth the time invested.

Once you have gathered the information needed, shop around! Ask a lot of questions, test ride a lot of bikes and then choose the bike your gut tells you you'll love. One sign that you have purchased the perfect bike for you is that you don't think about your bike when you are out riding—the bike is one with you and your experience on the road. You don't futz with your position in the saddle because it is simply correct. You don't worry about shifting problems or whether you will be able to come out of your pedals at the next stoplight, because your gears and pedals are perfectly adjusted for ease of use.

A poorly fitted bicycle, by contrast, will be uncomfortable to ride and potentially dangerous, serving as the cause of both major and minor injuries. If your bike fit is in question—or if you aren't sure what *to* question—ask around and get a referral to a reputable shop with a bike fit expert. Most quality shops should have at least one knowledgeable person on staff that can properly fit you to your bike.

HOW MUCH DO YOU WANT TO SPEND?

Purchasing a bike is similar to purchasing a car—the range of what you can spend is limitless, and the overall quality of your bike will partly depend on the price you pay.

Buying used is an excellent option because, just like a car, your bike depreciates significantly the second you ride it out of the shop. You can also take advantage of the not-so-smart-shopper who bought impulsively, only to let their several-thousand-dollar bike collect cobwebs in the garage.

The challenge with buying used is that it's tougher to find the "perfect" bike unless you have some time to shop around. Remember, if you have to compromise in any area when buying used, particularly in terms of fit, *don't* make the purchase.

You also don't need to commit to a high-end competitive bike right off the bat. I know many people who started cycling with a very basic bike and evolved their equipment as they matured as athletes. That is an excellent way to get your feet wet without spending a lot of money. Make sure you are going to enjoy the sport before you make a considerable investment.

If you do opt to buy, have your price range set before looking at the particular type of bike you are interested in using.

WHAT TYPE OF RIDING WILL YOU BE DOING?

Is your goal to do some century riding? Or are you more interested in bike touring, bike racing, or an occasional triathlon? If your answer is all of the above, then your puzzle just got a lot more complex. A bike set up for triathlon and one dialed for bike racing are two completely different animals.

However, if your focus is mainly on organized rides (with a triathlon thrown in for a fun challenge every now and again), you *can* work with one bike that meets your needs. Bike frames that are designed for all-around road riding tend to have relaxed seat tube, with angles in the

75–76-degree range. In general, this style of frame creates a relaxed climbing and descending experience as well as an overall comfortable ride.

WHAT TYPE OF FRAME MATERIAL DO YOU WANT?

For each type of frame material, there are countless cyclists who will argue why their preference is best. Often times, the budget you set for your new bike will automatically eliminate certain frame materials. Once you determine which materials are in your price range, you can start to examine the properties of each material, the ride qualities they offer, and then compare those to your preferences.

Aluminum is light and stiff—one of the stiffest frame materials out there. Aluminum frames don't have much flex, which allows for direct power transfer to the drive train. But all that stiffness can lead to body fatigue over a long haul or on bumpy roads. A heavier rider might do the best job subduing an aluminum bike's tendency to pop around on rough roads. If you are all about a quick ride on smooth roads while sprinting out of corners, seriously consider aluminum.

Carbon fiber is as light and comfortable as it gets. Carbon absorbs road shock so you don't have to, and is very popular for longer rides, rides over varying terrain, or for those with achy back problems. It is tough and stiff, but not as stiff as aluminum. Because of its shock-absorbing flex, carbon has been thought of as a poor sprinting or climbing-out-of-the-saddle bike, but much this depend on the design of the frame. The type of carbon, and the way it is put together (molded or lugged) can help define its power transfer properties (quality and feel varies with manufacturer). If you want a light, comfortable, high performance ride at a relatively reasonable price, carbon is for you.

Steel is the standard from which all bikes evolved, and some will ride a steel bike to the grave. It is durable, shock absorbent, and comfortable, and though not as quick as aluminum, it has an energetic feel. Steel is a pound or so heavier compared to titanium, carbon, and aluminum, but if you want a classic, all-around versatile feel on a tough frame, steel is for you.

Titanium has incredible qualities, and a price point to match. It is extremely light, shock absorbent, stiff in all riding situations, and durable. Titanium is unique in that it provides a consistent, quality ride for athletes of all weights. The downside is your titanium acquisition could cost you the equivalent of a down payment on a house in some areas of the United States.

WHAT ABOUT BIKE COMPONENTS?

Unless you are planning on putting your new frame together yourself as an off-season project, combining bits and pieces from different component manufacturers, you will probably be buying a bike that is fully built (with the exception of pedals). If you know from the start that you want to switch up any components, be sure to negotiate those changes into your original purchase. You'll save money on the ultimate bike price as well as mechanic fees for later changes.

Make sure you're heading out the door with the essentials:

- Bottle cage and water bottle

- A seat pack with a couple tubes

- Tire levers

- Patches

- Co_2 cartridges with valve adapter

- A small pump to carry along on your rides

Saddles: It will probably take some trial and error to get a saddle that works for you. Women's saddles are made a bit wider in the sit-bone area and many women swear by them, but I know a few women, myself included, who have had issues with the wider women's saddle putting too much pressure on the upper hamstring area. Many saddles have a center cutaway feature that minimizes compression to the pelvis and protects blood flow to the soft tissue of the crotch area, eliminating pain or numbness issues for both men and women. Ask your shop if they will let you test ride various saddles. There are many styles and designs to choose from, so there is no need to put up with an uncomfortable saddle. Find one that you don't even think about when you ride.

Aero bars: If you are planning to do even a couple of triathlons, get aero bars for your bike. Aero bars always seem to be that "I should have gotten these a long time ago!" piece of gear. Once you ride them and experience their comfort and speed advantage, you will never want to go back. Even if you are planning some century rides or bike touring, aero bars come in handy to take pressure off your hands over long distances. If they are set up appropriately, you will notice significant aerodynamic and comfort advantages immediately.

Tires: Your choice of tire width depends partly on your comfort level on the road. If you are new to road biking, start out with 23–25mm or wider. If you want a thinner, faster tire for racing, check your comfort level on a 20mm tire. Your tires are your connection to the ground, and it is important that they are well taken care of.

WHAT IS AVAILABLE TO BUY IN YOUR AREA?

If you've done your research and test ridden the items on your short list and know exactly which bike you want and what size you need, you can purchase your chosen bike anywhere it's available. This includes the internet, which may or may not be your best option. Sometimes, purchasing online can save you some money, but when making that internet purchase, consider the cost of shipping, having the bike built at a bike shop, and the cost of your initial tune-up. (Most shops will include the build and the first tweak with the price of the bike.)

The major advantage to using a local shop for your purchase is the relationship you build through that process. Finding and keeping a good mechanic and bike shop relationship is priceless. It may help you get your bike in for a quick pre-event tune up or prompt repair. Many shops will give repair preference to regular customers, which can help you get back out on the road more quickly.

Reputable shops, who sell mid- to high-end bikes, employ knowledgeable, experienced staff. If your local shop doesn't, or you don't feel comfortable with the person you are dealing with, ask to talk to someone else in the shop or go elsewhere. Although it's extremely helpful, you don't need to know a lot about bikes in order to make a solid purchase. However, you do need to have a positive feeling about the sales staff in order to develop a trusting relationship. If they're smart and they care, they will recognize the value in that relationship as well.

Developing a Relationship with Your Bike

n any sport, proper gear knowledge offers added familiarity and confidence to your time spent playing, and cycling is no different. Developing a relationship with your bicycle will increase your comfort level and efficiency on the roads. This includes understanding bike maintenance skills and how to take those skills out on the road while safely riding with cars, pedestrians, and other riders in close proximity.

BASIC MAINTENANCE

Part of understanding your bike is being able to perform basic maintenance while out riding. Learning to recognize tire problems and fixing them on the fly, like knowing how to change a flat, will increase your confidence in your cycling abilities.

For starters, take a flat tire changing class, usually offered by your local shop. Many of your riding buddies will have their own versions of proper flat tire changing, some of which may be inefficient; save yourself some trouble and don't learn any bad habits. Getting lessons on quick tire changing from a professional who does it regularly, then practicing what you've learned once a week until you can change your tire in several minutes or less, is the way to go. You *must* practice. Bring spare tubes on each ride and replace punctured tubes with new ones. Then, you can take your time at home patching the tube to use again while training.

While you're at the shop for your tire changing class, be sure to sign up for a bike maintenance class, which should cover tire and rim inspection, chain cleaning and lubing, and how to check the following:

- Handlebar stability

- Saddle and seat post stability

- Brakes and brake pad condition

- Crank arm stability

- Derailleur condition

- Whether your wheels are true (uniform when rotated) or wobbly

Once you learn these skills, be sure to do a weekly inspection of your bike. With the exception of chain cleaning and lubing, this will only take a few minutes once you've got it down.

All this being said, while it greatly enhances your relationship with your bike to be able to perform repairs, what is truly necessary is for you to be able to recognize problems and then report them accurately to your bike mechanic for repair.

Acquire and learn how to use:

- Allen wrenches (for all sizes of Allen bolts on your bike, plus your shoe cleats)

- Pedal wrench (always loosen backwards)

- Any other wrenches you may need (crank and headset)

- All-round bike grease for pedals and other bolts

- Chain tool and chain lube

- Extra flat tire changing gear (tubes, CO_2 cartridge and adapter, tire levers)

- Floor pump

Part of learning to love your bike is learning how to take care of it. It's fun! Plus, you can become the rider in your training group who has the knowledge needed to help your fellow riders.

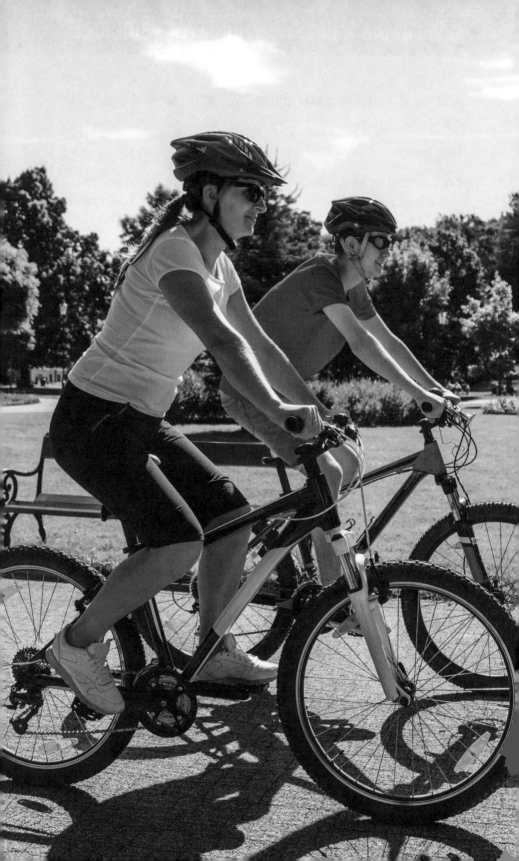

Road Etiquette for Group Riding

Knowing how to ride your bike on roads safely and respectfully is basic bike etiquette. Oftentimes the roads you ride, as well as the specific group you ride with, will further refine your riding process. In general, if you follow some fundamental guidelines, your road time will be much safer and more enjoyable.

Communicate distinctly and often. If you are riding in or near a group of other cyclists, don't assume that they know what you are going to do; tell them or signal to them. Say, "On your left" when passing, or, "Car back" when a car is overtaking your group. You should point to obstacles, holes, or problems in the road (like rocks or glass) so that riders behind you are aware. Create a hand signal for stopping and make sure that the riders you ride with understand what your signals mean.

Ride single file when on a road or bike path. Don't give cars any excuse to heckle you or drive too close. It's easy when in large numbers to fall prey to gang mentality and think you rule the road. However, you are required, just like motorists, to share the road. Live up to your end of that deal and give cyclists a better name out there.

Ride in a straight line. Be extremely aware of where you are and where the cyclists around you are at all times, but don't assume that others are doing the same. To best execute this process, always ride in a straight line and, if you plan to deviate in any way, communicate that you are doing so before you do it.

Use reflectors, a light, and a rear blinking light when riding in the dark, at daybreak, or dusk. Assume that you are invisible in the dark and use lighting that can be seen by all.

Always carry tools, your cell phone, and tire changing equipment. The more comfortable you feel riding around other moving entities on busy streets, the more you'll want to get out and ride. The more you practice these skills and help your training partners to acquire them as well, the more confident your cycling experiences will feel.

Fueling for the Long Ride

Having a very specific eating and drinking plan when heading out the door for a long day of riding is just as important as knowing your pacing plan for the ride or what type of shorts you'll need to wear to prevent chafing. This is important stuff and can take many training sessions to solidify.

There are three critical components to a training fueling plan: **calories, fluids,** and **electrolytes.**

The following guidelines will help you create your nutrition plan while keeping these components in check:

- Research indicates that endurance athletes need 150–400 calories per hour during activity. Consider factors such as exercise intensity and duration, fitness, and body size when determining how many calories you need to consume on a given day. Through practice, you'll be able to come up with an exact number that works for you, which you can then adapt as needed.

- The carbohydrates you consume should come primarily from glucose. It doesn't matter how you get these carbs—from drinks, gels, or bars. You must figure out which type or combination works best for you, and then consume the correct number of calories in whichever form suits you. Drink plain water with your gels or bars.

- Eat or drink your calories just like your car uses gas—steadily, not in one big gulp. Avoid taking in large quantities of calories infrequently as your body will not be able to assimilate more than 50–100 calories at a time. The result can be stomach problems or blood sugar issues as the food remains in the stomach. Take in 50–100 calories (along with some plain water) every 20–25 minutes during training. Do this consistently; Some people may need to set an alarm to remind them to eat at regular intervals.

- During exercise or at an event, drink 6–12 ounces (150–350 ml) of fluid every 20 minutes. Don't wait; start drinking shortly after you start. Personalize this quantity; the recommended amount may be too much or too little for you. Experiment with types and quantity and modify based on your stomach comfort, body size, and absorption, all the while making sure you are taking in plain water in addition to your chosen calories for optimal assimilation of calories from the stomach.

- Select sports drinks that include sodium or else consume something containing sodium, such as pretzels, chips, salty soup, etc. Sports drinks should also be 6–10 percent carbohydrate concentration for optimal absorption. This is a much lower concentration than is advised on the package of most drinks. If you enjoy it more concentrated, like most people, make sure you are cutting your sports drink with a couple swigs of plain water.

- Carbohydrates are your best source of fuel for training or events lasting 1–4 hours, but I have noticed that the majority of the people I coach desire some sources of protein and fat—especially in sessions lasting longer than a few hours. Too many carbs can be harsh on the stomach or palate; a bit of protein or fat can help settle the stomach and give you a sense of satisfaction. Don't force-feed yourself a carbs-only diet if it isn't working for your stomach or your psyche; experiment and allow yourself to come up with the protocol that works best for you.

GENERAL TERMS AND GUIDANCE

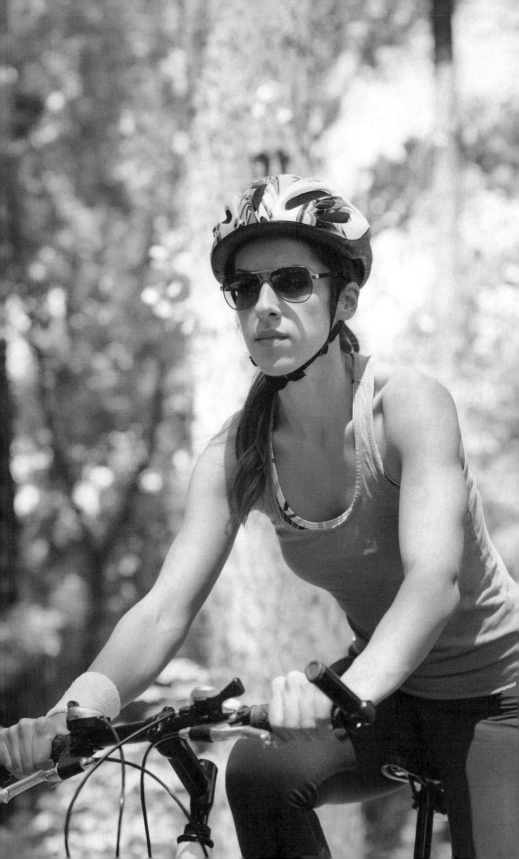

Essential Gear
for Cycling

While there are a lot of options available when outfitting yourself for cycling, there are definitely some essential pieces to have on hand to ensure safety and conduct proper maintenance.

Helmet: Always wear a helmet while riding your bike. You may be the best cyclist on the road, but the other riders and drivers around you may not be as competent or aware. You only need to witness one broken helmet to realize that it can save your life—or even better, protect you from the possibility of surviving a crash with serious brain damage. There are so many light, comfortable, and attractive helmets on the market, there is no excuse not to wear one.

For your helmet to work, you'll need to wear it low on your forehead so that the sides of the helmet can protect the fragile part of your skull on impact. Your chin strap should be comfortably snug. If you crash and your helmet takes a reasonable impact, throw it away and get a new one. Most lightweight helmets are *not* designed to withstand multiple crashes.

Floor Pump: Topping off your tires with a high-pressure pump each time you ride should be part of your regular bike maintenance process. It is common for your tires to lose 10 pounds or so of pressure after a few days. You can also use this pre-ride pump to do a quick check for any significant cuts or bulges in your tires that could cause problems on the road.

When inflating your tires, you may notice your tire has a number listed on the sidewall. This is the pressure rating, a number chosen for many reasons, most of which are not scientific. It may be chosen for legal or marketing reasons, and as such does not necessarily represent the amount of pressure you must have in your tires. For example, and despite using the same tire, a heavier rider will want more pressure than a lighter rider. An underinflated tire can cause rim or tire damage and pinch flats. If you know you are riding on smoother roads and you want to gain speed, reduce friction or the chance of pinch flats, or just want to create a quicker feel to your bike's steering, pump up your tires 10–30 PSI higher than what is stated on your tire. A smart rider will experiment with different tires and tire pressures and take note of what he enjoys and what feels comfortable.

Pedals and Shoes: Many people start out with a cycling shoe or fitness shoe combined with clips and straps, or flat pedals, and that's fine—for a start. But, if you know that you want to continue cycling as a regular addition to your fitness program, I recommend you opt for clipless pedals and work through the initial learning process right away. There are two types of riders: those who are going to fall over on their bike at a stop sign while trying to get out of their clipless pedals…and those who already have.

Once you get past the initial discomfort of clipping in and out, it will become second nature. Be patient with your progress and remember that the benefits you gain are worth the effort. Being connected to your pedals allows you to ride faster and more efficiently and truly become one with your bike.

If you have a pedal/shoe combination that makes it very difficult for you to come out of your pedals, see if your pedals can be adjusted or get different pedals that can. Most higher-end pedals have a smoother release mechanism that allows you to clip in and out without thinking about it. Look for a road pedal that allows you to clip in on both sides. Once you roll forward on your bike, you'll just place the cleated area of your shoe onto the pedal and press down—it's easy. Getting a lower-profile pedal will also give you some peace of mind if you decide to pedal through corners.

Road cycling shoes are designed with a stiff platform to best transfer the pressure from your foot to the pedal. Your road shoes should feel comfortable. If your shoe presses unduly on any particular part of your foot or repeatedly causes numb areas, try different shoes (or a different saddle). If you have a professional bike fit done, have the technician look at your shoes and feet, how they are placed over the pedals, and how they track when you pedal, as inconsistency in any of these areas can cause foot issues on your bike.

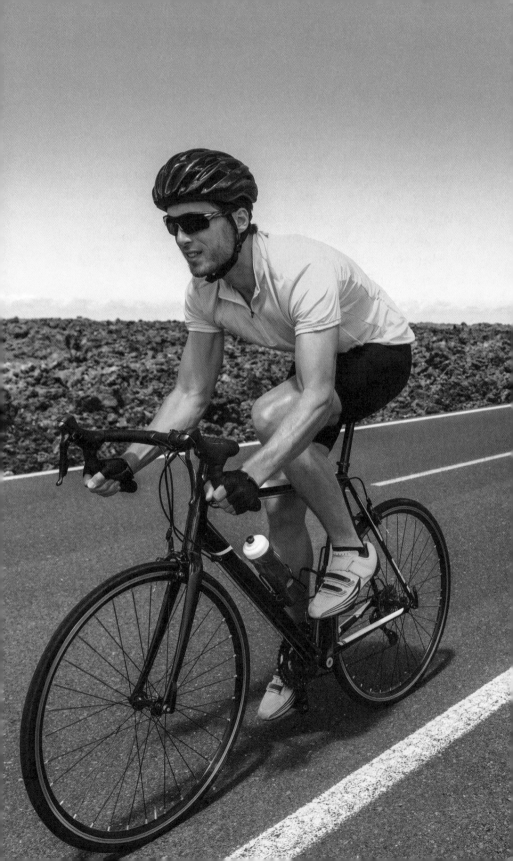

Bicycle Accessories

Bike shorts and other clothing: If you are new to cycling or still have sit bone or crotch issues on your bike, try some new bike shorts or a new bike saddle (seat). Cycling shorts (for training) should be comfortable and offer more padding and zero chafing. Do not wear underwear with your bike shorts. The extra pressure can chafe or create discomfort; cycling shorts are made to be worn alone.

There are many other clothing accessories you can purchase to make your cycling experiences functional, comfortable, and fun. Evaluate the weather in which you usually ride and make your clothing choices accordingly. Consider wearing gloves for comfort and to protect your hands.

As an example, I live in an area that oftentimes has morning fog prior to things getting sunny and warm. For longer rides, even in the summertime, I always carry a windbreaker that I can wad up as small as my fist, in case it gets a bit chilly. You can get bike jerseys with pockets (long, short, or no-sleeves), tights, and leg or arm warmers (my favorites). Shop around, look for sales, and enjoy outfitting yourself for your new sport!

Bicycle computers: Depending on the bike computer you purchase, its functions may include GPS (global positioning system), an odometer, trip distance, auto start/stop functions, a stopwatch, a clock, tire size memory, heart rate monitor functions, a timer, an alarm, cadence, altimeter, temperature, and current, maximum, and average speed.

At minimum, your computer should provide information on how far you went, how long it took, and what your average speed was. This is helpful data for you to learn more about your cycling progress, as well as note areas for improvement. Just like a heart rate monitor, a bike computer of any kind is not a prerequisite but is a helpful tool in refining your skills as an endurance athlete.

Heart rate monitor: Heart rate monitors are a helpful training tool as they aid you in executing each workout at the desired intensity level. Many bike computers also have built-in heart rate monitors. If you do purchase a heart rate monitor, you'll need to shop around to find a monitor you feel comfortable using and that has all the functions you need to suit your training program. At minimum, get a monitor that has a heart rate function, along with time and stopwatch settings. The extras you'll want will depend on how detailed you wish to become in your training program. Do some research and choose a monitor that will best aid you.

Helpful Workout Terminology

Ab crunches (abdominal crunches): Lie on the ground, a bench, or an exercise ball with your feet flat. Place your hands either across your chest or behind your head. Lift your chin and shoulders directly upward toward the sky. Hold for one second. Release your shoulders back to the ground.

Brick: A brick workout is a workout combining two or more disciplines executed one after another without a break in between. In triathlons, this usually entails a bike/run workout.

Build: Progressively increase the speed of the interval.

Crank arm: The arm that attaches the pedal to the bike.

Cross-training: Engaging in two or more sports or types of exercise within your total fitness program.

Derailleur: Mechanisms that move the chain, in the act of shifting gears on a bike.

Descend the set: Progressively increase the speed of each interval in a set.

Evens: 2nd, 4th, 6th, etc. intervals within a set.

Fartlek: Fartlek, or speed-play, is typically a whimsical and spontaneous, run or bike speed session—you increase your pace when and how much you wish, as you go. For the fartlek workouts outlined in this book, either use the guidelines offered within each workout to approximate your efforts within each session, or just go out and bike or run as you feel for the allotted time.

Fastest average: The fastest pace you can average for the given set and rest interval.

Fastest time: Your fastest time for the designated interval.

Hill extension: Repetition of an incline followed by maintained intensity for a designated period over and beyond the top of the incline.

Hill repeats: Repetitions of high-intensity work followed by periods of rest or low activity. Done on an incline.

Intervals: Repetitions of high-speed and high-intensity work followed by periods of rest or low activity.

Odds: 1st, 3rd, 5th, etc. intervals within a set.

Periodize: Modulating volume and intensity of training over time to both stimulate gains and allow recovery.

Pick up: Gradually building your speed up to a fast pace over 100 meters or a designated time.

Side shuffle lunges: Step to the side then do a squat with your back straight. After you squat fully, push yourself up to standing while at the same time shuffling your feet and taking a step to the side. This is similar to a skipping motion to the side. Finish the shuffle with your feet apart in preparation to squat and shuffle again.

Spinning: When a cyclist turns the pedals around lightly and quickly, while in a low (easy) gear.

Stride or bike stride: Gradually building your speed from a moderate to a fast pace over the allotted distance or time.

Tempo riding: Tempo runs include a designated period of time(s) in which you run at a specific and consistent pace. The goal is to run the designated tempo time, sustaining the allotted pace.

Time: For the workouts in this book, ":30" or "30 min." is understood to mean 30 minutes, and "1:10" means 1 hour and 10 minutes.

Training effect: The cardiovascular and structural "advancement" that the body attains through training, specifically the effect that training has on an athlete's body physiologically, structurally, and cardiovascularly. In order to gain training effect, an athlete needs both training stress and recovery/rest.

Training level variations: Move between given levels (for example L1–L2, L3–L4, etc.) during the designated time given, generally by hovering between them. See the Training Levels Chart on page 38 for more details.

Walking lunges: Take long walking steps and lunge down to 90 degrees at the knee joint with each step. Keep your upper body upright and use your arms for balance as needed.

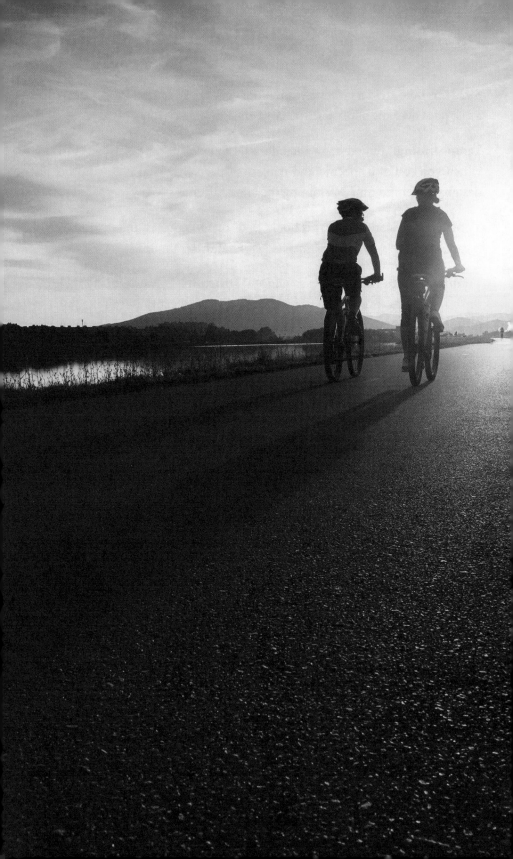

Training Principles for Cycling

There are many skills that you will need to learn in order to become a safe and competent cyclist. Some of these include climbing, descending, cornering, shifting, and braking. In order to fine-tune your ability in each area, I recommend that you seek the help of a patient and qualified cyclist or coach who is willing to spend some time with you on the bike. The more skilled you become in each of these areas, the better cyclist you will be and the more you will enjoy riding your bike.

GEARING AND SPINNING

When an athlete gets on a bike for the first time, their tendency is to push the pedals at 40–60 revolutions per minute (RPMs). This low turnover rate is not only inefficient, but it puts stress on the knees and muscles and over time can set you up for injury. To learn to effectively turn the pedals at a natural and efficient cadence, cyclists incorporate spinning into their riding routine.

Spinning is a technique where a rider turns the pedals around lightly and quickly while in a low (easy) gear, keeping RPMs at around 85–100. You can count your RPMs, or better yet use a bike computer with cadence capabilities to determine your RPMs. While spinning, focus on technique; speed and power will come later. Spinning requires you to exert pressure down and then back with one pedal, while releasing the pressure and/or pulling up on the opposite pedal. While spinning perfect circles, relax your upper body as much as possible and focus on this leg and hip activity. The objective is to spin fluidly and quickly while maintaining openness and stillness in the hip area.

Each gear combination on your bike allows the bike to move forward a set number of inches with one pedal stroke. The bigger the gear, the farther you travel with each revolution. The more power you exert on that big gear, the quicker it covers its corresponding inches. And most importantly, the more refined your spin with each turn of the pedals, the more chance your power will be transferred with perfect efficiency.

If you are only pushing down on each pedal to generate speed, you are missing a significant component to your pedal stroke, and you will likely make the mistake of continuing to push down when the pedal is in the recovery phase. In a flawless spin, one pedal should be pushing down while the other is pulling up. Since the pulling up phase takes enormous strength and refinement of technique, concentrate first on releasing pressure on the pedal in recovery. Once you have mastered a consistent release of pressure, you can then move into developing the pulling up motion.

The power being transferred from your body to the bike comes predominantly from your quads, hamstrings, calves, and gluteus muscles. With relaxed yet stable ankles, your hip and knee joints flex and extend, but your hips remain basically stable on your saddle. If you are rocking back and forth on your saddle, then you either have muscular tightness that is not allowing you to spin fluidly, your saddle is too high, or you need to refine your spin.

Spending time each week to improve your spin technique is time well spent. Use your easy recovery rides or portions of your longer training sessions spinning. Have a friend or bike fit technician video tape you from the front, side, and behind to review your spin and note ways to improve. Your goal may be to slowly increase gears to increase speed and power, but never compromise the fluidity of your spin.

PACING

One of the essential skills of endurance riding is figuring out your optimal pace for a given distance. This takes time and effort and requires continual evaluation and refinement.

Even pacing requires you to have either an understanding of what heart rate you should be hitting for a certain distance, or a solid inner pace clock that allows you to target your effort objective. One way to gain knowledge of your inner pace clock is to use the *Borg Scale of Perceived Exertion* (see page 40). The Borg Scale is an excellent way to gauge your level of intensity in training and competition without a heart rate monitor (see Training Levels).

If you are doing your first 100K organized ride and your first objective is to complete the distance, you may decide that hitting an effort level of around 11–14 on the Borg Scale would be prudent—especially if you are unsure of your fitness.

As you test your pacing capabilities in training, you will gain a solid knowledge of what you are capable of for a given distance on the bike (though this may change as your fitness increases). Whichever effort level you choose on the bike, the key is to hit it evenly. Riding hard, then easy, then hard will needlessly burn up fuel, decrease your average speed, and kill motivation faster than riding at a steady, solid effort throughout the event.

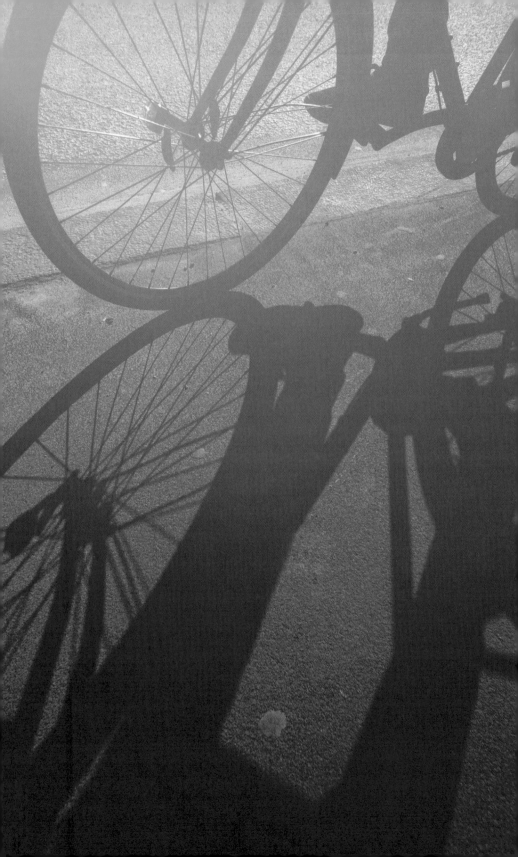

Training Levels

Each of the following sections describes your workout using training levels in the Training Levels Chart on page 38. These are described by:

- What it is used for

- One's "perceived exertion," using the Borg Perceived Exertion chart on page 40

- Corresponding heart rate (HR) range (see below)

Heart rate (HR) range is shown as an assigned "% of max" number. This number designates an HR range relative to your maximum HR. For example, 80% of max is 80% of your maximum HR. You can choose which method of evaluating your intensity level suits you; however, in order to use the "% of max" numbers within each level, you must know your max HR.

If you are not currently using a heart rate monitor or you have not tested for your max HR, use the Training Levels Chart on page 38 to decipher your workout efforts via how a level is used or by your perceived exertion (using the Borg Perceived Exertion Scale on page 40). It is important for you to become familiar with these workout levels and how they feel for you.

If you have a heart rate monitor and you know your max HR (*only* by taking a max HR test, *not* by using a formula), you can use your monitor to establish training intensity on the Training Levels Chart. Otherwise, use the additional information on the chart to establish your workout levels.

TRAINING LEVELS CHART

(See the Borg Perceived Exertion scale on page 40)

Level 1: Recovery

- *Used for*: Recovery, warm-up, cool-down, and baseline endurance

- *Perceived Exertion (PE)*: 9-10; you can talk easily, effort is extremely easy

- *HR Range*: 65-75% of max

Level 2: Aerobic

- *Used for*: Improving aerobic, or oxygen utilization capacity, warm-up, cool-down, and longer training and races

- *Perceived Exertion (PE)*: 11–13; conversations are comfortable, effort is moderate to easy

- *HR Range*: 75–80% of max

Level 3: High-End Aerobic to Low Anaerobic

- *Used for*: Improving lactate system, intervals, hills, tempo training, and long-to- moderate distance training and races

- *Perceived Exertion (PE)*: 14–15; short conversations are possible, effort is moderate to challenging

- *HR Range*: 80–85% of max

Level 4: Lactate or Anaerobic Threshold

- *Used for*: Improving ability to mobilize lactate for longer periods, intervals, hills, and moderate- to short-distance training and races

- *Perceived Exertion (PE)*: 16–18; difficult to speak, effort is challenging to difficult

- *HR Range*: 85-90% of max

Level 5: Sub-Maximum to Maximum Effort*

- *Used for*: Training fast twitch muscles to develop power, strength, and speed; intervals; and sprint training and events

- *Perceived Exertion (PE)*: 19–20; breathing is labored, effort is very difficult

- *HR Range*: 90-100% of max

*__Maximum HR__ is pre-set, or genetic, and can be determined optimally through a max heart rate test. Maximum HR will decline with age. We cannot train our max HR to become higher, but we can train to be better at taking a max HR test.

BORG PERCEIVED EXERTION (PE) SCALE

The Borg Perceived Exertion (PE) Scale gives you an idea of how hard exercise feels. Use the below scale to aid your efforts to work within the corresponding training levels designated for each workout in your training program:

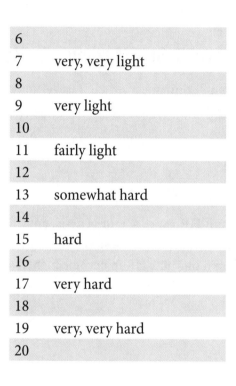

6	
7	very, very light
8	
9	very light
10	
11	fairly light
12	
13	somewhat hard
14	
15	hard
16	
17	very hard
18	
19	very, very hard
20	

Stretching for Endurance Athletes

Your weekly plan should include daily stretching. Stretching is useful for injury prevention, maintaining range of motion, and helping you connect with areas of your body that need attending to. If you already incorporate a stretching or yoga program into your training routine, continue to execute that program each day. If you are not currently stretching, start performing the following stretches daily:

Standing Spinal Twist: Stand with your hands clasping a tree, fence, or wall. Slowly turn your lower body to the left, away from the fence, while maintaining your upper body position toward the fence. Keep your spin straight and long. Do the same on the right side.

Standing Side Stretch: Stand with your feet shoulder-width apart. Raise both arms to the side and clasp them overhead while maintaining a straight spine and hips. Extend your clasped hands toward the sky and bend from the hips, slightly to the right side. With your arms continually extended, move through your center and bend to the other side.

Standing Hamstring Stretch: Place one ankle on a raised object (the height of the object will be dependent on how flexible your hamstrings are). Only raise your leg to a height that allows you to feel a gentle stretch. Keep your pelvis in a straight line with your spine (do not tilt your pelvis). You may feel the stretch while remaining upright. If so, continue standing upright. If you need more of a stretch, lean slightly forward while keeping your spine long and straight.

Calf Stretch: Stand about three feet from a wall or fence, with your feet shoulder-width apart, flat on the ground, and toes pointing forward. Put your hands on the fence with your arms straight for support. Lean your hips forward with a soft bend in your knees to stretch your calves. You can also do this stretch focusing on one leg at a time for more focused effect.

Standing Quad Stretch: Stand on one foot with one hand on an object for balance. Hold the top of your foot with the opposite hand and raise the heel of the lifted foot to the buttocks (or as close as comfortably possible), stretching your quadriceps. Keep both knees close together with your spine and hips in a straight line throughout. Change legs and repeat on the other side.

CYCLING
WORKOUTS

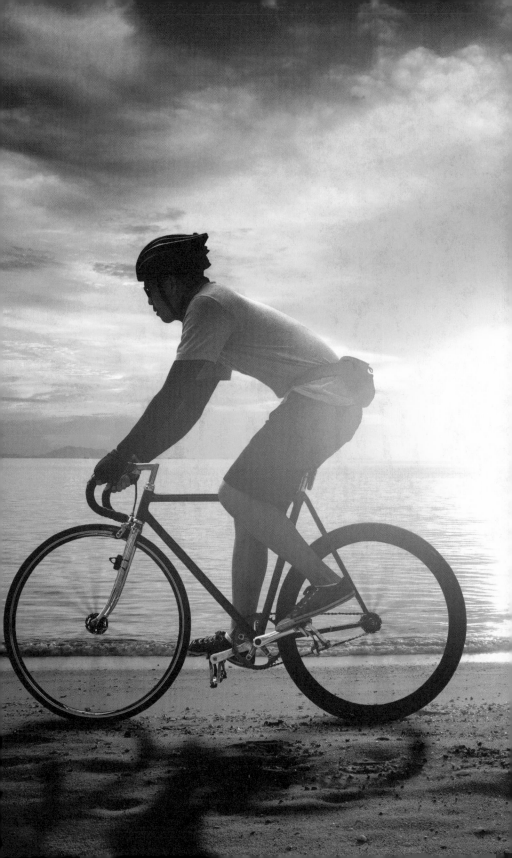

Fitness Program: Cycling for Fitness and Fun

:30 to 2:30 per Day

PROGRAM GUIDELINES
Who

This program is for those who ride 2–4 days per week (sometimes more, sometimes less) and whose cycling sessions vary in length but generally last between 20–90 minutes—sometimes more. This program is intended for those just getting started in their cycling program, who have been a cyclist for a few months, or who have a limited amount of time to devote to their fitness program but want to ensure they get a productive week of training in. You may or may not have experience with organized rides but would like to take your training to the next level.

What and How

This program is your map for each week of bike training. Your week incorporates: recovery, high intensity options (intervals, tempo), hill training, and long/long fartlek training sessions. This program comes with multiple options within each session category. You can change sessions each week as you wish, mixing them up to keep your training fun and challenging. Sessions are listed in each category with increasing difficulty. I recommend starting at the top of the list and making your way down as your fitness increases.

If you have been cycling 2–4 days per week, I recommend you continue doing so for a few weeks before you increase the quantity of bike sessions per week. If you have been cycling 3–4 or more sessions per week, continue to do so while adding 1–2 bike sessions after a couple of months. Take additional recovery sessions or rest days, as needed.

Rules

- Use the guidelines in your program to plug in training sessions on given days.

- Do not do high intensity or hill sessions on back-to-back days. Take a recovery day between each of these sessions.

- Do each workout at the prescribed training level. For example, do your recovery sessions at L1–L2, which is a very easy effort. This will help you get the most out of your more challenging workouts and allow for your best overall training effect.

- After 2–3 weeks of executing this program, do one active recovery week in which you decrease the overall time and intensity of each session by 20–30%. The following week you can jump back up to a full week. Repeat this pattern with 2–3 weeks of prescribed training, followed by an easier week. This is a means to periodize your program and is necessary to get the full effect from your training.

Strength Training

If you have done consistent strength training prior to going into this program and you have the time available, continue to execute your strength training routine while incorporating the strength and core exercises shown in this program. If you have not been doing any strength work, execute the strength and core exercises as designated in this program, while using the above rules as a guide.

FITNESS PROGRAM: CYCLING FOR FITNESS AND FUN :30 TO 2 HOURS 30 MINUTES PER DAY

Day 1

STRETCH :15

REST DAY

Day 2

STRETCH :15

BIKE SESSION: Choose one workout from one of these lists: INTERVALS or TEMPO

Walking Lunges: 3x10

Side Shuffle Lunges: 3x10

Push-ups: 3x10 (full plank or knees-down push-ups, whichever you can do while maintaining a straight torso)

Ab crunches: 40

Day 3: RECOVERY

STRETCH :15

REST DAY, CROSS-TRAIN, or BIKE :30 (L1–L2)

Day 4

STRETCH :15

BIKE SESSION*: Choose one workout from this list: HILLS.

Walking Lunges: 3x10

Side Shuffle Lunges: 3x10

Push-ups: 3x10 (full plank or knees-down push-ups, whichever you can do while maintaining a straight torso)

Ab crunches: 40

* If you are still feeling tired from your Day 2 session, do Day 5 RECOVERY workout today and do your HILLS session on Day 5.

Day 5: RECOVERY

STRETCH :15

REST DAY or CROSS-TRAIN

Day 6

STRETCH :15

REST DAY or BIKE :30 (L1–L3)

Day 7

STRETCH :15

BIKE SESSION: Choose one workout from the LONG or LONG/FARTLEK session list. Start with the distance you are currently doing with your long ride, then gradually work your way down the list each week. After 2–3 weeks of executing your long ride on this day, do one active recovery week in which you decrease the overall time and intensity of this session by 20–30%.

Day 2 SESSION

Choose *one* workout from *one* of the below session categories.

INTERVALS:
30 minutes to 45 minutes

Choose a flat route for this workout.

DAY 2 INTERVALS

INTERVAL 1
<u>BIKE :30 (L1–L4)</u>

Warm up at L1–L2 for :05

2x30 second pick-ups with 1 minute at L2 between each

3x1 minute at L3–L4 with 1 minute between each

Cool down the remaining time at L1–L2

L1 - Level 1: Recovery; **L2** - Level 2: Aerobic; **L3** - Level 3: High-End Aerobic to Low Anaerobic;
L4 - Level 4: Lactate or Anaerobic Threshold; **L5** - Level 5: Sub-Maximum to Maximum Effort

INTERVAL 2
BIKE :35 (L1–L4)

Warm up at L1–L2 for :05

4x30 second pick-ups with 1 minute at L2 between each

4x2 minutes at L3–L4 with 1 minute at L2 between each

Cool down the remaining time at L1–L2

L1 - Level 1: Recovery; **L2** - Level 2: Aerobic; **L3** - Level 3: High-End Aerobic to Low Anaerobic;
L4 - Level 4: Lactate or Anaerobic Threshold; **L5** - Level 5: Sub-Maximum to Maximum Effort

DAY 2 INTERVALS

INTERVAL 3
<u>BIKE :40 (L1–L4)</u>

Warm up at L1–L2 for :05

4x30 second pick-ups with 1 minute at L2 between each

3x2 minutes at L4 with 1:30 minutes at L2 between each

2x3 minutes at L3–L4 with 2 minutes at L2 between each

Cool down the remaining time at L1–L2

L1 - Level 1: Recovery; L2 - Level 2: Aerobic; L3 - Level 3: High-End Aerobic to Low Anaerobic;
L4 - Level 4: Lactate or Anaerobic Threshold; L5 - Level 5: Sub-Maximum to Maximum Effort

INTERVAL 4
BIKE :40 (L1–L4)

Warm up at L1–L2 for :05

6x1 minute pick-ups with 30 seconds at L2 between each

1, 2, 3, 2, 1 minute at L4. Ride at L2 between each for the same amount of time as the interval prior.

Cool down the remaining time at L1–L2

L1 - Level 1: Recovery; L2 - Level 2: Aerobic; L3 - Level 3: High-End Aerobic to Low Anaerobic; L4 - Level 4: Lactate or Anaerobic Threshold; L5 - Level 5: Sub-Maximum to Maximum Effort

DAY 2 INTERVALS

INTERVAL 5
BIKE :45 (L1–L4)

Warm up at L1–L2 for :05

4x30 second pick-ups with 30 seconds at L2 between each

4x4 minutes at L3–L4 with 3 minutes at L2 between each

Cool down the remaining time at L1–L2

L1 - Level 1: Recovery; **L2** - Level 2: Aerobic; **L3** - Level 3: High-End Aerobic to Low Anaerobic; **L4** - Level 4: Lactate or Anaerobic Threshold; **L5** - Level 5: Sub-Maximum to Maximum Effort

INTERVAL 6
BIKE :45 (L1–L4)

Warm up at L1–L2 for :05

2x1 minute pick-ups with 30 seconds at L2 between each

1, 2, 3, 4, 3, 2, 1 minute at L4. Ride at L2 between each for the same amount of time as the interval prior.

Cool down the remaining time at L1–L2

L1 - Level 1: Recovery; **L2** - Level 2: Aerobic; **L3** - Level 3: High-End Aerobic to Low Anaerobic; **L4** - Level 4: Lactate or Anaerobic Threshold; **L5** - Level 5: Sub-Maximum to Maximum Effort

TEMPO:
30 minutes to 50 minutes

These sessions can be done anywhere and on any type of terrain. Tempo rides include a designated period of time in which you ride at a specific and consistent pace. The goal is to ride the designated tempo time, sustaining the allotted pace.

TEMPO 1
BIKE :30 (L1–L3)

Warm up at L1–L2 for :08

5 minutes at L3
4 minutes at L2
5 minutes at L3

Cool down the remaining time at L1–L2

L1 - Level 1: Recovery; L2 - Level 2: Aerobic; L3 - Level 3: High-End Aerobic to Low Anaerobic;
L4 - Level 4: Lactate or Anaerobic Threshold; L5 - Level 5: Sub-Maximum to Maximum Effort

TEMPO 2
BIKE :30 (L1–L4)

Warm up at L1–L2 for :07

8 minutes at L3
3 minutes at L2
3 minutes at L3–L4

Cool down the remaining time at L1–L2

L1 - Level 1: Recovery; L2 - Level 2: Aerobic; L3 - Level 3: High-End Aerobic to Low Anaerobic; L4 - Level 4: Lactate or Anaerobic Threshold; L5 - Level 5: Sub-Maximum to Maximum Effort

DAY 2 TEMPO

TEMPO 3
BIKE :35 (L1–L4)

Warm up at L1–L2 for :10

15 minutes at L3–L4

Cool down the remaining time at L1–L2

L1 - Level 1: Recovery; L2 - Level 2: Aerobic; L3 - Level 3: High-End Aerobic to Low Anaerobic; L4 - Level 4: Lactate or Anaerobic Threshold; L5 - Level 5: Sub-Maximum to Maximum Effort

TEMPO 4
BIKE :40 (L1–L4)

DAY 2 TEMPO

Warm up at L1–L2 for :10

7 minutes at L3
3 minutes at L2
8 minutes at L4

Cool down the remaining time at L1–L2

L1 - Level 1: Recovery; L2 - Level 2: Aerobic; L3 - Level 3: High-End Aerobic to Low Anaerobic; L4 - Level 4: Lactate or Anaerobic Threshold; L5 - Level 5: Sub-Maximum to Maximum Effort

DAY 2 TEMPO

TEMPO 5
BIKE :45 (L1–L4)

Warm up at L1–L2 for :10

10 minutes at L3

11 minutes at L3–L4

Cool down the remaining time at L1–
    L2

L1 - Level 1: Recovery; **L2** - Level 2: Aerobic; **L3** - Level 3: High-End Aerobic to Low Anaerobic;
L4 - Level 4: Lactate or Anaerobic Threshold; **L5** - Level 5: Sub-Maximum to Maximum Effort

TEMPO 6
BIKE :50 (L1–L4)

Warm up at L1–L2 for :10

15 minutes at L3
5 minutes at L2
10 minutes at L4

Cool down the remaining time at L1–L2

L1 - Level 1: Recovery; L2 - Level 2: Aerobic; L3 - Level 3: High-End Aerobic to Low Anaerobic;
L4 - Level 4: Lactate or Anaerobic Threshold; L5 - Level 5: Sub-Maximum to Maximum Effort

Day 4 SESSION

Choose *one* workout from *one* of
the below session categories.

HILLS:
30 minutes to 50 minutes

Hill workouts include; increasing pace on hills within a ride, hill repeats, and sustained hill efforts. If you have more time for this workout and you have been consistently doing hill training prior to taking on this program, add 1–2 more hill efforts within the workout.

DAY 4 HILLS

HILLS 1
<u>BIKE :30 (L1–L4)</u>

Choose a hilly BIKE route that includes at least 3 hills that take 1 minute or less to ride up

Warm up at L1–L2 for :10 on flatter terrain prior to arriving at your first hill effort

When you come to a hill ride it at L3–L4. Continue your ride to the next hill at L2, then repeat the L3–L4 effort on the next incline.

Once 4 hills are completed cool down the remaining time at L1–L2

L1 - Level 1: Recovery; **L2** - Level 2: Aerobic; **L3** - Level 3: High-End Aerobic to Low Anaerobic; **L4** - Level 4: Lactate or Anaerobic Threshold; **L5** - Level 5: Sub-Maximum to Maximum Effort

HILLS 2
BIKE :30 (L1–L4)

Warm up at L1–L2 for :10 on flat terrain

Choose a hill that takes you 20-30 seconds to ride up

Ride this hill 5x at L4. Between each coast slowly to the bottom, take an additional 30 seconds recovery before executing your next incline.

Cool down the remaining time at L1–L2

L1 - Level 1: Recovery; L2 - Level 2: Aerobic; L3 - Level 3: High-End Aerobic to Low Anaerobic;
L4 - Level 4: Lactate or Anaerobic Threshold; L5 - Level 5: Sub-Maximum to Maximum Effort

DAY 4 HILLS

HILLS 3
BIKE :35 (L1–L4)

Warm up at L1–L2 for :10 on flat
terrain

Choose a hill that takes you 30-40
seconds to ride up

Ride this hill 6x at L3–L4. Coast
slowly to the bottom of the hill
then immediately execute your
next incline.

Cool down the remaining time at L1–
L2

L1 - Level 1: Recovery; **L2** - Level 2: Aerobic; **L3** - Level 3: High-End Aerobic to Low Anaerobic;
L4 - Level 4: Lactate or Anaerobic Threshold; **L5** - Level 5: Sub-Maximum to Maximum Effort

HILLS 4
BIKE :40 (L1–L4)

Warm up at L1–L2 for :10 on flat terrain

Choose a hill that takes you 30-40 seconds to ride up

Ride this hill 7x at L4, extending your effort for an additional 10 seconds over the top and as the terrain flattens out. Coast slowly to the bottom of the hill then immediately execute your next hill-extension.

Cool down the remaining time at L1–L2

L1 - Level 1: Recovery; L2 - Level 2: Aerobic; L3 - Level 3: High-End Aerobic to Low Anaerobic; L4 - Level 4: Lactate or Anaerobic Threshold; L5 - Level 5: Sub-Maximum to Maximum Effort

DAY 4 HILLS

HILLS 5
BIKE :45 (L1–L4)

Warm up at L1–L2 for :15 on flat terrain

Choose a long gradual hill that is 1 mile or further in length

Start up the hill riding 30 seconds at L4, continue up the hill riding easily for 1 minute. Repeat this process 6x as you continue making your way up the hill. If you reach the top of the hill prior to finishing the set, turn around and execute recovery on a down slope before riding up again.

Cool down the remaining time at L1–L2

L1 - Level 1: Recovery; L2 - Level 2: Aerobic; L3 - Level 3: High-End Aerobic to Low Anaerobic;
L4 - Level 4: Lactate or Anaerobic Threshold; L5 - Level 5: Sub-Maximum to Maximum Effort

HILLS 6
BIKE :50 (L1–L4)

Warm up at L1–L2 for :15 on flat terrain

Choose a long gradual hill that is 1 mile or further in length

Start up the hill riding 40 seconds at L4, continue up the hill riding easily for 1 minute. Repeat this process 8x as you continue making your way up the hill. If you reach the top of the hill prior to finishing the set, turn around and execute recovery on a down slope before riding up again.

Cool down the remaining time at L2–L3

L1 - Level 1: Recovery; **L2** - Level 2: Aerobic; **L3** - Level 3: High-End Aerobic to Low Anaerobic; **L4** - Level 4: Lactate or Anaerobic Threshold; **L5** - Level 5: Sub-Maximum to Maximum Effort

Day 7 SESSION

Choose *one* workout below.

LONG OR LONG/FARTLEK: 1 hour to 2 hours 30 minutes

The LONG BIKE is your longest ride of the week. Fartlek, or speed-play, is typically a whimsical and sponta- neous speed session—you increase your pace when and how much you wish, as you go. Use the guidelines to approximate your efforts within each LONG/FARTLEK session. You do not have to execute the speed increases in the order they are listed. You can add them in as you wish.

DAY 7 LONG/FARTLEK

LONG/FARTLEK 1
BIKE 1:00

Warm up at L1–L2 for :15

Within the rest of the ride do the following when you wish:

3 speed increases for: 1 minute between telephone poles or trees, or a similar length/ distance. Ride a similar length of time/distance at L2 between each.

2 speed increase for: 2 minutes or a half mile in length. Use your watch or choose an object en route as a finish point.

BIKE the remaining time at L2–L3

L1 - Level 1: Recovery; **L2** - Level 2: Aerobic; **L3** - Level 3: High-End Aerobic to Low Anaerobic; **L4** - Level 4: Lactate or Anaerobic Threshold; **L5** - Level 5: Sub-Maximum to Maximum Effort

LONG/FARTLEK 2
BIKE 1:15

Warm up at L1–L2 for :15

Within the rest of the ride do the following when you wish:

2 speed increases for: 1 minute between telephone poles or trees, or a similar length/ distance. Ride a similar length of time/distance at L2 between each.

2 speed increases for: 2 minutes or a half mile in length. Use your watch or choose an object en route as a finish point. Take as much time as you wish riding at L2 between each.

1 speed increase for: 3 minutes or a mile in length. Use your watch or

L1 - Level 1: Recovery; **L2** - Level 2: Aerobic; **L3** - Level 3: High-End Aerobic to Low Anaerobic; **L4** - Level 4: Lactate or Anaerobic Threshold; **L5** - Level 5: Sub-Maximum to Maximum Effort

DAY 7 LONG/FARTLEK

choose an object en route as a finish point. Take as much time as you wish riding at L2 prior to your next speed play.

BIKE the remaining time at L2–L3

L1 - Level 1: Recovery; **L2** - Level 2: Aerobic; **L3** - Level 3: High-End Aerobic to Low Anaerobic;
L4 - Level 4: Lactate or Anaerobic Threshold; **L5** - Level 5: Sub-Maximum to Maximum Effort

LONG 3
BIKE 1:30 (L1–L4)

Warm up at L1–L2 for :25

BIKE L2–L3 for :10
BIKE L3–L4 for :05
BIKE L4 for :05

BIKE the remaining time at L2–L3

L1 - Level 1: Recovery; **L2** - Level 2: Aerobic; **L3** - Level 3: High-End Aerobic to Low Anaerobic;
L4 - Level 4: Lactate or Anaerobic Threshold; **L5** - Level 5: Sub-Maximum to Maximum Effort

DAY 7 LONG/FARTLEK

LONG 4
BIKE 1:45 (L1–L4)

Warm up at L1–L2 for :25

BIKE L3 for :10
BIKE L4 for :05
BIKE L2 for :10
BIKE L4 for :05

BIKE the remaining time at L2–L3

L1 - Level 1: Recovery; L2 - Level 2: Aerobic; L3 - Level 3: High-End Aerobic to Low Anaerobic; L4 - Level 4: Lactate or Anaerobic Threshold; L5 - Level 5: Sub-Maximum to Maximum Effort

LONG/FARTLEK 5
BIKE 1:45

Warm up at L1–L2 for :25

Within the rest of the ride do the following when you wish:

10 speed increases, each less than 1 minute or approximately a half mile. Use your watch or choose an object en route as a finish point.

Take as much time as you wish at L2 between each while making sure you have completed all 10 when your watch hits 1:35.

BIKE the remaining time at L2–L3

L1 - Level 1: Recovery; **L2** - Level 2: Aerobic; **L3** - Level 3: High-End Aerobic to Low Anaerobic;
L4 - Level 4: Lactate or Anaerobic Threshold; **L5** - Level 5: Sub-Maximum to Maximum Effort

LONG/FARTLEK 6
<u>BIKE 2:00</u>

Warm up at L1–L2 for :25

Within the rest of the ride do the following when you wish:

4 speed increases for: 30 seconds between telephone poles or trees, or a similar length/ distance. Ride a similar length of time/distance at L2 between each.

4 speed increases for: 2 minutes or approximately a half of a mile. Use your watch or choose an object en route as a finish point.

L1 - Level 1: Recovery; **L2** - Level 2: Aerobic; **L3** - Level 3: High-End Aerobic to Low Anaerobic; **L4** - Level 4: Lactate or Anaerobic Threshold; **L5** - Level 5: Sub-Maximum to Maximum Effort

Take as much time as you wish at L2 between each while making sure you have completed all speed increases when your watch hits 1:45.

BIKE the remaining time at L2–L3

DAY 7 LONG/FARTLEK

L1 - Level 1: Recovery; **L2** - Level 2: Aerobic; **L3** - Level 3: High-End Aerobic to Low Anaerobic;
L4 - Level 4: Lactate or Anaerobic Threshold; **L5** - Level 5: Sub-Maximum to Maximum Effort

DAY 7 LONG/FARTLEK

LONG 7
BIKE 2:00 (L1–L4)

Warm up at L1–L2 for :25

BIKE L2–L3 for :25
BIKE L4 for :10

BIKE the remaining time at L2–L3

L1 - Level 1: Recovery; L2 - Level 2: Aerobic; L3 - Level 3: High-End Aerobic to Low Anaerobic; L4 - Level 4: Lactate or Anaerobic Threshold; L5 - Level 5: Sub-Maximum to Maximum Effort

LONG 8
BIKE 2:00 (L1–L4)

Warm up at L1–L2 for :25

BIKE L2–L3 for :15
BIKE L3–L4 for :10

BIKE the remaining time at L2–L3

DAY 7 LONG/FARTLEK

L1 - Level 1: Recovery; **L2** - Level 2: Aerobic; **L3** - Level 3: High-End Aerobic to Low Anaerobic;
L4 - Level 4: Lactate or Anaerobic Threshold; **L5** - Level 5: Sub-Maximum to Maximum Effort

DAY 7 LONG/FARTLEK

LONG/FARTLEK 9
BIKE 2:15

Warm up at L1–L2 for :25

Within the rest of the ride do the following when you wish:

8 speed increases for: 1 minute between telephone poles or trees, or a similar length/ distance. Ride a similar length of time/distance at L2 between each.

3 speed increase for: 2 minutes or a half mile in length. Use your watch or choose an object en route as a finish point. Take as much time as you wish riding at L2 between each.

BIKE the remaining time at L2–L3

L1 - Level 1: Recovery; **L2** - Level 2: Aerobic; **L3** - Level 3: High-End Aerobic to Low Anaerobic;
L4 - Level 4: Lactate or Anaerobic Threshold; **L5** - Level 5: Sub-Maximum to Maximum Effort

LONG/FARTLEK 10
BIKE 2:15

Warm up at L1–L2 for :25

Within the rest of the ride do the following when you wish:

4 speed increases for: 1 minute between telephone poles or trees, or a similar length/ distance. Take as much time as you wish riding at L2 between each.

4 speed increases for: 2 minutes or a half mile in length. Use your watch or choose an object en route as a finish point. Take as much time as you wish riding at L2 between each.

L1 - Level 1: Recovery; **L2** - Level 2: Aerobic; **L3** - Level 3: High-End Aerobic to Low Anaerobic; **L4** - Level 4: Lactate or Anaerobic Threshold; **L5** - Level 5: Sub-Maximum to Maximum Effort

DAY 7 LONG/FARTLEK

1 speed increase for: 3 minutes or a mile in length. Use your watch or choose an object en route as a finish point.

BIKE the remaining time at L2–L3

L1 - Level 1: Recovery; **L2** - Level 2: Aerobic; **L3** - Level 3: High-End Aerobic to Low Anaerobic; **L4** - Level 4: Lactate or Anaerobic Threshold; **L5** - Level 5: Sub-Maximum to Maximum Effort

LONG 11
BIKE 2:15 (L1–L4)

Warm up at L1–L2 for :25

BIKE L2–L3 for :10
BIKE L3–L4 for :05
BIKE L4 for :05

BIKE the remaining time at L2–L3

L1 - Level 1: Recovery; L2 - Level 2: Aerobic; L3 - Level 3: High-End Aerobic to Low Anaerobic;
L4 - Level 4: Lactate or Anaerobic Threshold; L5 - Level 5: Sub-Maximum to Maximum Effort

LONG 12
BIKE 2:30 (L1–L4)

DAY 7 LONG/FARTLEK

Warm up at L1–L2 for :30

BIKE L3 for :10
BIKE L4 for :05
BIKE L3 for :10
BIKE L4 for :05

BIKE the remaining time at L2–L3

L1 - Level 1: Recovery; L2 - Level 2: Aerobic; L3 - Level 3: High-End Aerobic to Low Anaerobic;
L4 - Level 4: Lactate or Anaerobic Threshold; L5 - Level 5: Sub-Maximum to Maximum Effort

LONG/FARTLEK 13
BIKE 2:30

Warm up at L1–L2 for :30

Within the rest of the BIKE do the following when you wish:

10 speed increases, each less than 1 minute or approximately 300 yards. Use your watch or choose an object en route as a finish point.

Take as much time as you wish between each while making sure you have completed all 10 when your watch hits 2:00.

BIKE the remaining time at L2–L3

DAY 7 LONG/FARTLEK

L1 - Level 1: Recovery; **L2** - Level 2: Aerobic; **L3** - Level 3: High-End Aerobic to Low Anaerobic; **L4** - Level 4: Lactate or Anaerobic Threshold; **L5** - Level 5: Sub-Maximum to Maximum Effort

DAY 7 LONG/FARTLEK

LONG/FARTLEK 14
BIKE 2:30

Warm up at L1–L2 for :30

Within the rest of the BIKE do the following when you wish:

8 speed increases for: 30 seconds between telephone poles or trees, or a similar length/ distance. Take as much time as you wish riding at L2 between each.

4 speed increases for: 2 minutes or approximately a half a mile. Use your watch or choose an object en route as a finish point.

L1 - Level 1: Recovery; **L2** - Level 2: Aerobic; **L3** - Level 3: High-End Aerobic to Low Anaerobic; **L4** - Level 4: Lactate or Anaerobic Threshold; **L5** - Level 5: Sub-Maximum to Maximum Effort

Take as much time as you wish between each at L2 while making sure you have completed all speed increases when your watch hits 2:00.

BIKE the remaining time at L2–L3

DAY 7 LONG/FARTLEK

L1 - Level 1: Recovery; L2 - Level 2: Aerobic; L3 - Level 3: High-End Aerobic to Low Anaerobic; L4 - Level 4: Lactate or Anaerobic Threshold; L5 - Level 5: Sub-Maximum to Maximum Effort

DAY 7 LONG/FARTLEK

LONG 15
BIKE 2:30 (L1–L4)

Warm up at L1–L2 for :30

BIKE L2–L3 for :25
BIKE L4 for :05
BIKE L2–L3 for :25
BIKE L4 for :05

BIKE the remaining time at L2–L3

L1 - Level 1: Recovery; **L2** - Level 2: Aerobic; **L3** - Level 3: High-End Aerobic to Low Anaerobic; **L4** - Level 4: Lactate or Anaerobic Threshold; **L5** - Level 5: Sub-Maximum to Maximum Effort

LONG 16
BIKE 2:30 (L1–L4)

Warm up at L1–L2 for :30

BIKE L2–L3 for :15
BIKE L3–L4 for :15

BIKE the remaining time at L2–L3

DAY 7 LONG/FARTLEK

L1 - Level 1: Recovery; L2 - Level 2: Aerobic; L3 - Level 3: High-End Aerobic to Low Anaerobic; L4 - Level 4: Lactate or Anaerobic Threshold; L5 - Level 5: Sub-Maximum to Maximum Effort

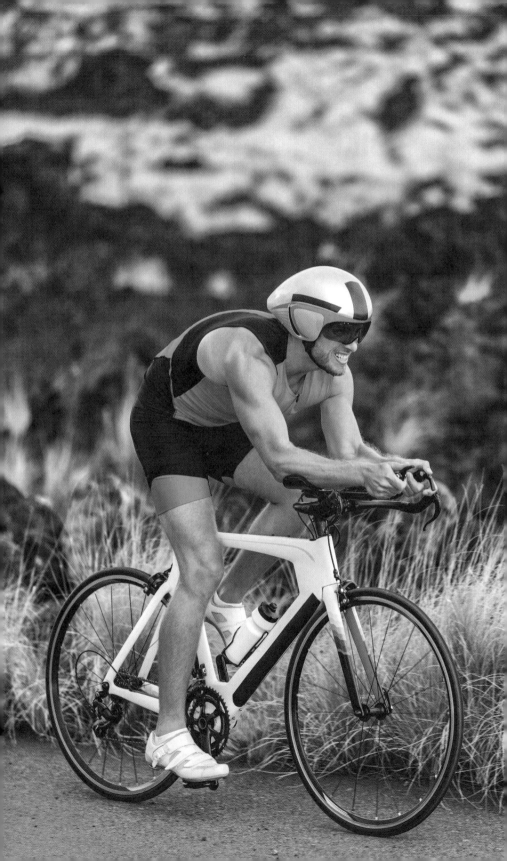

Build Program:
Train for a 50 Mile
or 100K Ride

40 Minutes to 3 Hours 30 Minutes

PROGRAM GUIDELINES

Who

This program is for those who ride an average of 3–5 days per week and whose cycling sessions vary in length but generally last between 40 minutes and 2 hours (or sometimes more). Use this program if you have been riding for at least a few months or have a specific amount of time to devote to your fitness program and want to ensure you get in a challenging week of training. You may or may not have experience with organized cycling events but would like to take your training to the next level. You have your eyes set on riding a 50 mile or 100K event.

What and How

This program is your map for each week of bike training. Your week will incorporate: recovery, high intensity options (intervals, tempo), hill training and long/long fartlek training sessions. This program comes with multiple options within each session category. You can change sessions each week as you wish, mixing them up to keep your training fun and challenging. Sessions are listed within each category with increasing difficulty. I recommend starting at the top of the list and making your way down as your fitness increases.

If you have been biking 3–4 days per week, I recommend you continue doing so for a few weeks before you increase the quantity of sessions per week. If you have been cycling 4 or more sessions per week, continue to do so while adding 1–2 bike sessions after several weeks. Take additional recovery sessions or rest days, as needed.

Rules

- Use the guidelines in your program to plug in training sessions on given days.

- Do not do high intensity and hill sessions on back-to-back days. Take a recovery day between each of these sessions.

- Do each workout at the prescribed training level. For example, do your recovery sessions at L1–L2, which is a very easy effort. This will help you get the most out of your more challenging workouts and allow for your best overall training effect.

- After 2–3 weeks of executing this program, do one active recovery week in which you decrease the overall time and intensity of each session by 20–30%. The following week you can jump back up to a full week. Repeat this pattern with 2–3 weeks of prescribed training, followed by an easier week. This is a means to periodize your program and is necessary to get the full effect from your training.

Strength Training

If you have done consistent strength training prior to going into this program and you have the time available, continue to execute your strength training routine while adding in the strength and core exercises shown in this program. If you have not been doing any strength work, execute the strength and core exercises as designated in this program, while using the above rules as a guide.

BUILD PROGRAM:
40 MINUTES TO 3 HOUR 30 MINUTES PER DAY

Day 1

STRETCH :15

REST DAY

Day 2

STRETCH :15

BIKE SESSION: Choose one workout from one of these lists: INTERVALS or TEMPO

Walking Lunges: 3x15

Side Shuffle Lunges: 3x15

Push-ups: 3x15 (full plank or knees-down push-ups, whichever you can do while maintaining a straight torso)

Ab crunches: 60

Day 3: RECOVERY

STRETCH :15

REST DAY, CROSS-TRAIN, or BIKE :40 (L1–L2)

Day 4

STRETCH :15

BIKE SESSION*: Choose one workout from this list: HILLS

Walking Lunges: 3x15

Side Shuffle Lunges: 3x15

Push-ups: 3x15 (full plank or knees-down push-ups, whichever you can do what maintaining a straight torso)

Ab crunches: 60

*If you are still feeling tired from your Day 2 session, do Day 5 RECOVERY workout today and do your HILL session on Day 5.

Day 5: RECOVERY

STRETCH :15

REST DAY, CROSS-TRAIN, or BIKE :45 - (L1–L2)

Day 6

STRETCH :15

BIKE :50 (L1–L3)

Day 7

STRETCH :15

BIKE SESSION: Choose one workout from the LONG or LONG/FARTLEK session list. Start with the distance you are currently doing with your long ride, then gradually work your way down the list each week. After 2–3 weeks of executing your long ride on this day, do one active recovery week in which you decrease the overall time and intensity of this session by 20–30%.

Day 2 SESSION

Choose *one* workout from *one* of the
below session categories.

INTERVALS:
45 minutes to 1 hour

Choose a flat route for this workout.

INTERVAL 1
BIKE :45 (L1–L4)

Warm up at L1–L2 for :10

3x30 second pick-ups with 1 minute at L2 between each

1, 2, 2, 1 minute at L3–L4 with 2 minutes at L2 between each

Cool down the remaining time at L1–L2

L1 - Level 1: Recovery; L2 - Level 2: Aerobic; L3 - Level 3: High-End Aerobic to Low Anaerobic; L4 - Level 4: Lactate or Anaerobic Threshold; L5 - Level 5: Sub-Maximum to Maximum Effort

INTERVAL 2
BIKE :45 (L1–L4)

Warm up at L1–L2 for :10

2x30 second pick-ups with 1 minute at L2 between each

6x2 minutes at L4 with 1:30 minutes at L2 between each

2x30 second pick-ups with 1 minute at L2 between each

Cool down the remaining time at L1–L2

L1 - Level 1: Recovery; L2 - Level 2: Aerobic; L3 - Level 3: High-End Aerobic to Low Anaerobic; L4 - Level 4: Lactate or Anaerobic Threshold; L5 - Level 5: Sub-Maximum to Maximum Effort

DAY 2 INTERVALS

INTERVAL 3
BIKE :50 (L1–L4)

Warm up at L1–L2 for :10

2x30 second pick-ups with 1 minute at L2 between each

2x2 minutes at L4 with 1:30 minutes at L2 between each

2x4 minutes at L3 with 3 minutes at L2 between each

2x2 minutes at L4 with 1:30 minutes at L2 between each

Cool down the remaining time at L1–L2

INTERVAL 4
BIKE :50 (L1–L4)

Warm up at L1–L2 for :10

2x1 minute pick-ups with 30 seconds at L2 between each

1, 2, 3, 3, 3, 2, 1 minute at L4. Ride at L2 between each for the same amount of time as the interval prior.

Cool down the remaining time at L1–L2

L1 - Level 1: Recovery; **L2** - Level 2: Aerobic; **L3** - Level 3: High-End Aerobic to Low Anaerobic; **L4** - Level 4: Lactate or Anaerobic Threshold; **L5** - Level 5: Sub-Maximum to Maximum Effort

DAY 2 INTERVALS

INTERVAL 5
BIKE 1:00 (L1–L4)

Warm up at L1–L2 for :10

4x1 minute pick-ups with 30 seconds at L2 between each

4x4 minutes at L3–L4 with 3 minutes at L2 between each

Cool down the remaining time at L1–L2

L1 - Level 1: Recovery; L2 - Level 2: Aerobic; L3 - Level 3: High-End Aerobic to Low Anaerobic; L4 - Level 4: Lactate or Anaerobic Threshold; L5 - Level 5: Sub-Maximum to Maximum Effort

INTERVAL 6
BIKE 1:00 (L1–L4)

Warm up at L1–L2 for :10

4x1 minute pick-ups with 30 seconds at L2 between each

1, 2, 3, 4, 3, 2, 1 minute at L4. Ride at L2 between each for the same amount of time as the interval prior.

Cool down the remaining time at L1–L2

L1 - Level 1: Recovery; **L2** - Level 2: Aerobic; **L3** - Level 3: High-End Aerobic to Low Anaerobic; **L4** - Level 4: Lactate or Anaerobic Threshold; **L5** - Level 5: Sub-Maximum to Maximum Effort

TEMPO:
40 minutes to 1 hour

These sessions can be done anywhere and on any type of terrain. Tempo bike sessions include a designated period of time in which you ride at a specific and consistent pace. The goal is to ride the designated tempo time, sustaining the allotted pace.

DAY 2 TEMPO

TEMPO 1
BIKE :40 (L1–L3)

Warm up at L1–L2 for :10

8 minutes at L3
2 minutes at L2
8 minutes at L3

Cool down the remaining time at L1–L2

L1 - Level 1: Recovery; L2 - Level 2: Aerobic; L3 - Level 3: High-End Aerobic to Low Anaerobic; L4 - Level 4: Lactate or Anaerobic Threshold; L5 - Level 5: Sub-Maximum to Maximum Effort

TEMPO 2
<u>BIKE :40 (L1–L4)</u>

Warm up at L1–L2 for :10

10 minutes at L3
2 minutes at L2
5 minutes at L3–L4

Cool down the remaining time at L1–L2

L1 - Level 1: Recovery; L2 - Level 2: Aerobic; L3 - Level 3: High-End Aerobic to Low Anaerobic; L4 - Level 4: Lactate or Anaerobic Threshold; L5 - Level 5: Sub-Maximum to Maximum Effort

TEMPO 3
<u>BIKE :50 (L1–L3)</u>

Warm up at L1–L2 for :10

15 minutes at L3

Cool down the remaining time at L1–L2

L1 - Level 1: Recovery; **L2** - Level 2: Aerobic; **L3** - Level 3: High-End Aerobic to Low Anaerobic; **L4** - Level 4: Lactate or Anaerobic Threshold; **L5** - Level 5: Sub-Maximum to Maximum Effort

TEMPO 4
BIKE :50 (L1–L4)

Warm up at L1–L2 for :10

13 minutes at L3
2 minutes at L2
5 minutes at L4

**Cool down the remaining time at L1–
      L2**

L1 - Level 1: Recovery; L2 - Level 2: Aerobic; L3 - Level 3: High-End Aerobic to Low Anaerobic;
L4 - Level 4: Lactate or Anaerobic Threshold; L5 - Level 5: Sub-Maximum to Maximum Effort

DAY 2 TEMPO

TEMPO 5
BIKE 1:00 (L1–L3)

Warm up at L1–L2 for :10

10 minutes at L3
10 minutes at L3–L4

Cool down the remaining time at L1–
   L2

L1 - Level 1: Recovery; L2 - Level 2: Aerobic; L3 - Level 3: High-End Aerobic to Low Anaerobic;
L4 - Level 4: Lactate or Anaerobic Threshold; L5 - Level 5: Sub-Maximum to Maximum Effort

TEMPO 6
BIKE 1:00 (L1–L4)

DAY 2 TEMPO

Warm up at L1–L2 for :10

13 minutes at L3
2 minutes at L2
5 minutes at L4

**Cool down the remaining time at L1–
L2**

L1 - Level 1: Recovery; L2 - Level 2: Aerobic; L3 - Level 3: High-End Aerobic to Low Anaerobic;
L4 - Level 4: Lactate or Anaerobic Threshold; L5 - Level 5: Sub-Maximum to Maximum Effort

Day 4 SESSION

Choose *one* workout from *one* of the
below session categories.

HILLS:
40 minutes to 1 hour

Hill workouts include; increasing pace on hills within a ride, hill repeats, and sustained hill efforts. If you have more time for this workout and you have been consistently doing hill training prior to taking on this program, add 1-2 more hill efforts within the workout.

DAY 4 HILLS

HILLS 1
BIKE :40 (L1–L4)

Choose a hilly BIKE route that includes at least 4-6 hills that take 1 minute or less to ride up

Warm up at L1–L2 for :10 on flatter terrain prior to arriving at your first hill effort

When you come to a hill ride it at L3–L4. Continue your ride to the next hill at L2, then repeat the L3–L4 effort on the next incline.

Once 4-6 hills are completed cool down the remaining time at L1–L2

L1 - Level 1: Recovery; **L2** - Level 2: Aerobic; **L3** - Level 3: High-End Aerobic to Low Anaerobic; **L4** - Level 4: Lactate or Anaerobic Threshold; **L5** - Level 5: Sub-Maximum to Maximum Effort

HILLS 2
<u>BIKE :40 (L1–L4)</u>

DAY 4 HILLS

Warm up at L1–L2 for :10 on flat
   terrain

Choose a hill that takes you 45
   seconds to 1 minute to ride up

BIKE this hill 6x at L4. Between each
   coast slowly to the bottom,
   take an additional 30 seconds
   recovery before executing your
   next incline.

Cool down the remaining time at L1–
   L2

L1 - Level 1: Recovery; **L2** - Level 2: Aerobic; **L3** - Level 3: High-End Aerobic to Low Anaerobic;
L4 - Level 4: Lactate or Anaerobic Threshold; **L5** - Level 5: Sub-Maximum to Maximum Effort

DAY 4 HILLS

HILLS 3
<u>BIKE :50 (L1–L4)</u>

Warm up at L1–L2 for :10 on flat
  terrain

Choose a hill that takes you 1:30
  minutes to ride up

BIKE this hill 6x at L3–L4. Coast
  slowly to the bottom of the hill
  and immediately execute your
  next incline.

Cool down the remaining time at L1–
  L2

L1 - Level 1: Recovery; L2 - Level 2: Aerobic; L3 - Level 3: High-End Aerobic to Low Anaerobic;
L4 - Level 4: Lactate or Anaerobic Threshold; L5 - Level 5: Sub-Maximum to Maximum Effort

HILLS 4
BIKE :50 (L1–L4)

Warm up at L1–L2 for :10 on flat terrain

Choose a hill that takes you 1:30 minutes to ride up

BIKE this hill 6x at L4, extending your effort for an additional 10 seconds over the top and as the terrain flattens out. Coast slowly to the bottom of the hill and immediately execute your next hill-extension.

Cool down the remaining time at L1–L2

L1 - Level 1: Recovery; L2 - Level 2: Aerobic; L3 - Level 3: High-End Aerobic to Low Anaerobic; L4 - Level 4: Lactate or Anaerobic Threshold; L5 - Level 5: Sub-Maximum to Maximum Effort

DAY 4 HILLS

HILLS 5
BIKE 1:00 (L1–L4)

Warm up at L1–L2 for :10 on flat
terrain

Choose a long gradual hill that is 1
mile or further in length

Start up the hill riding 1 minute at L4,
continue up the hill for 1 minute
at L2. Repeat this process 7x as
you continue making your way
up the hill.

If you cannot maintain an L2 effort
during recovery, then extend the
recovery interval.

L1 - Level 1: Recovery; L2 - Level 2: Aerobic; L3 - Level 3: High-End Aerobic to Low Anaerobic;
L4 - Level 4: Lactate or Anaerobic Threshold; L5 - Level 5: Sub-Maximum to Maximum Effort

If you reach the top of the hill prior to finishing the set, then turn around and execute recovery on a down slope before riding up again.

Cool down the remaining time at L1–L2

DAY 4 HILLS

L1 - Level 1: Recovery; **L2** - Level 2: Aerobic; **L3** - Level 3: High-End Aerobic to Low Anaerobic; **L4** - Level 4: Lactate or Anaerobic Threshold; **L5** - Level 5: Sub-Maximum to Maximum Effort

DAY 4 HILLS

HILLS 6
BIKE 1:00 (L1–L4)

Warm up at L1–L2 for :10 on flat
  terrain

Choose a hill that takes you 2 minutes
  to ride up

BIKE this hill 7x at L4, extending
  your effort for an additional 10
  seconds over the top and as the
  terrain flattens out. Coast slowly
  to the bottom of the hill and
  immediately execute your next
  hill-extension.

Cool down the remaining time at L1–
  L2

L1 - Level 1: Recovery; L2 - Level 2: Aerobic; L3 - Level 3: High-End Aerobic to Low Anaerobic;
L4 - Level 4: Lactate or Anaerobic Threshold; L5 - Level 5: Sub-Maximum to Maximum Effort

Day 7 SESSION

Choose *one* workout below.

LONG OR LONG/FARTLEK:
2 hours to 3 hour 30 minutes

The long bike is your longest ride of the week. Fartlek, or speed-play, is typically a whimsical and spontaneous speed session—you increase your pace when and how much you wish, as you go. Use the guidelines to approximate your efforts within each long/fartlek session. You do not have to execute the speed increases in the order they are listed. You can add them in as you wish.

DAY 7 LONG/FARTLEK

LONG/FARTLEK 1
BIKE 2:00

Warm up at L1–L2 for :20

Within the rest of the ride do the following when you wish:

3 speed increases for: 1 minute between telephone poles or trees, or a similar length/ distance. Take a similar length of time/distance at L2 between each.

4 speed increases for: 2 minutes or a half mile in length. Use your watch or an object en route as a finish point. Take as much time as you wish between each.

BIKE the remaining time at L2–L3

L1 - Level 1: Recovery; L2 - Level 2: Aerobic; L3 - Level 3: High-End Aerobic to Low Anaerobic; L4 - Level 4: Lactate or Anaerobic Threshold; L5 - Level 5: Sub-Maximum to Maximum Effort

LONG/FARTLEK 2
BIKE 2:00

Warm up at L1–L2 for :20

Within the rest of the ride do the following when you wish:

3 speed increases for: 1 minute between telephone poles or trees, or a similar length/ distance. Take a similar length of time/distance at L2 between each.

2 speed increases for: 2 minutes or a half mile in length. Use your watch or an object en route as a finish point.

2 speed increases for: 3 minutes or a mile in length. Use your watch or an object en route as a finish point.

DAY 7 LONG/FARTLEK

L1 - Level 1: Recovery; **L2** - Level 2: Aerobic; **L3** - Level 3: High-End Aerobic to Low Anaerobic; **L4** - Level 4: Lactate or Anaerobic Threshold; **L5** - Level 5: Sub-Maximum to Maximum Effort

DAY 7 LONG/FARTLEK

Take as much time as you wish between each.

BIKE the remaining time at L2–L3

LONG 3
BIKE 2:15 (L1–L4)

Warm up at L1–L2 for :25

BIKE L2–L3 for :20
BIKE L3–L4 for :05
BIKE L4 for :05

BIKE the remaining time at L2–L3

L1 - Level 1: Recovery; **L2** - Level 2: Aerobic; **L3** - Level 3: High-End Aerobic to Low Anaerobic;
L4 - Level 4: Lactate or Anaerobic Threshold; **L5** - Level 5: Sub-Maximum to Maximum Effort

LONG 4
BIKE 2:15 (L1–L4)

DAY 7 LONG/FARTLEK

Warm up at L1–L2 for :25

BIKE L3 for :10
BIKE L4 for :05
BIKE L3 for :10
BIKE L4 for :05

BIKE the remaining time at L2–L3

L1 - Level 1: Recovery; L2 - Level 2: Aerobic; L3 - Level 3: High-End Aerobic to Low Anaerobic;
L4 - Level 4: Lactate or Anaerobic Threshold; L5 - Level 5: Sub-Maximum to Maximum Effort

LONG/FARTLEK 5
<u>BIKE 2:30</u>

Warm up at L1–L2 for :30

Within the rest of the ride do the following when you wish:

10 speed increases, each less than 1 minute or approximately a half mile. Use your watch or an object en route as a finish point.

Take as much time as you wish between each.

BIKE the remaining time at L2–L3

L1 - Level 1: Recovery; **L2** - Level 2: Aerobic; **L3** - Level 3: High-End Aerobic to Low Anaerobic; **L4** - Level 4: Lactate or Anaerobic Threshold; **L5** - Level 5: Sub-Maximum to Maximum Effort

DAY 7 LONG/FARTLEK

LONG/FARTLEK 6
BIKE 2:30

Warm up at L1–L2 for :30

Within the rest of the ride do the
following when you wish:

4 speed increases for: 30 seconds
between telephone poles or
trees, or a similar length/
distance. Take a similar length
of time/distance at L2 between
each.

3 speed increases for: 4 min or
approximately one mile. Use your
watch or an object en route as a
finish point.

Take as much time as you wish
between each.

BIKE the remaining time at L2–L3

L1 - Level 1: Recovery; L2 - Level 2: Aerobic; L3 - Level 3: High-End Aerobic to Low Anaerobic;
L4 - Level 4: Lactate or Anaerobic Threshold; L5 - Level 5: Sub-Maximum to Maximum Effort

LONG 7
BIKE 2:45 (L1–L4)

Warm up at L1–L2 for :35

BIKE L2–L3 for :35
BIKE L4 for :10

BIKE the remaining time at L2–L3

L1 - Level 1: Recovery; L2 - Level 2: Aerobic; L3 - Level 3: High-End Aerobic to Low Anaerobic;
L4 - Level 4: Lactate or Anaerobic Threshold; L5 - Level 5: Sub-Maximum to Maximum Effort

DAY 7 LONG/FARTLEK

LONG 8
BIKE 2:45 (L1–L4)

Warm up at L1–L2 for :35

BIKE L2–L3 for :25

BIKE L3–L4 for :10

BIKE the remaining time at L2–L3

L1 - Level 1: Recovery; L2 - Level 2: Aerobic; L3 - Level 3: High-End Aerobic to Low Anaerobic; L4 - Level 4: Lactate or Anaerobic Threshold; L5 - Level 5: Sub-Maximum to Maximum Effort

LONG/FARTLEK 9
BIKE 3:00

Warm up at L1–L2 for :40

Within the rest of the ride do the following when you wish:

3 speed increases for: 1 minute between telephone poles or trees, or a similar length/ distance. Take a similar length of time/distance at L2 between each.

6 speed increases for: 2 minutes or a half mile in length. Use your watch or an object en route as a finish point. Take as much time as you wish between each.

BIKE the remaining time at L2–L3

L1 - Level 1: Recovery; L2 - Level 2: Aerobic; L3 - Level 3: High-End Aerobic to Low Anaerobic;
L4 - Level 4: Lactate or Anaerobic Threshold; L5 - Level 5: Sub-Maximum to Maximum Effort

LONG/FARTLEK 10
BIKE 3:00

Warm up at L1–L2 for :40

Within the rest of the ride do the following when you wish:

3 speed increases for: 1 minute, between telephone poles or trees, or a similar length/distance. Take a similar length of time/distance at L2 between each.

2 speed increases for: 2 minutes or a half mile in length. Use your watch or an object en route as a finish point.

3 speed increases for: 3 minutes or a mile in length. Use your watch or an object en route as a finish point.

L1 - Level 1: Recovery; L2 - Level 2: Aerobic; L3 - Level 3: High-End Aerobic to Low Anaerobic; L4 - Level 4: Lactate or Anaerobic Threshold; L5 - Level 5: Sub-Maximum to Maximum Effort

Take as much time as you wish between each.

BIKE the remaining time at L2–L3

L1 - Level 1: Recovery; **L2** - Level 2: Aerobic; **L3** - Level 3: High-End Aerobic to Low Anaerobic; **L4** - Level 4: Lactate or Anaerobic Threshold; **L5** - Level 5: Sub-Maximum to Maximum Effort

DAY 7 LONG/FARTLEK

LONG 11
BIKE 3:15 (L1–L4)

Warm up at L1–L2 for :40

BIKE L2–L3 for :20

BIKE L3–L4 for :05

BIKE L4 for :05

BIKE the remaining time at L2–L3

L1 - Level 1: Recovery; L2 - Level 2: Aerobic; L3 - Level 3: High-End Aerobic to Low Anaerobic; L4 - Level 4: Lactate or Anaerobic Threshold; L5 - Level 5: Sub-Maximum to Maximum Effort

LONG 12
<u>BIKE 3:15 (L1–L4)</u>

Warm up at L1–L2 for :45

BIKE L3 for :10

BIKE L4 for :05

BIKE L3 for :10

BIKE L4 for :05

BIKE the remaining time at L2–L3

L1 - Level 1: Recovery; **L2** - Level 2: Aerobic; **L3** - Level 3: High-End Aerobic to Low Anaerobic;
L4 - Level 4: Lactate or Anaerobic Threshold; **L5** - Level 5: Sub-Maximum to Maximum Effort

LONG/FARTLEK 13
BIKE 3:30

Warm up at L1–L2 for :45

Within the rest of the ride do the following when you wish:

10 speed increases, each less than 1 minute or approximately a half mile. Use your watch or an object en route as a finish point.

Take as much time as you wish between each.

BIKE the remaining time at L2–L3

L1 - Level 1: Recovery; **L2** - Level 2: Aerobic; **L3** - Level 3: High-End Aerobic to Low Anaerobic;
L4 - Level 4: Lactate or Anaerobic Threshold; **L5** - Level 5: Sub-Maximum to Maximum Effort

LONG/FARTLEK 14
BIKE 3:30

Warm up at L1–L2 for :45

Within the rest of the ride do the following when you wish:

4 speed increases for: 30 seconds between telephone poles or trees, or a similar length/distance. Take a similar length of time/distance at L2 between each.

3 speed increases for: 4 min or approximately a mile. Use your watch or an object en route as a finish point.

Take as much time as you wish between each.

BIKE the remaining time at L2–L3

L1 - Level 1: Recovery; L2 - Level 2: Aerobic; L3 - Level 3: High-End Aerobic to Low Anaerobic; L4 - Level 4: Lactate or Anaerobic Threshold; L5 - Level 5: Sub-Maximum to Maximum Effort

LONG 15
<u>BIKE 3:30 (L1–L4)</u>

DAY 7 LONG/FARTLEK

Warm up at L1–L2 for :45

BIKE L2–L3 for :35
BIKE L4 for :05

BIKE the remaining time at L2–L3

L1 - Level 1: Recovery; L2 - Level 2: Aerobic; L3 - Level 3: High-End Aerobic to Low Anaerobic; L4 - Level 4: Lactate or Anaerobic Threshold; L5 - Level 5: Sub-Maximum to Maximum Effort

LONG 16
<u>BIKE 3:30 (L1–L4)</u>

Warm up at L1–L2 for :45

BIKE L2–L3 for :25
BIKE L3–L4 for :10

BIKE the remaining time at L2–L3

DAY 7 LONG/FARTLEK

L1 - Level 1: Recovery; L2 - Level 2: Aerobic; L3 - Level 3: High-End Aerobic to Low Anaerobic;
L4 - Level 4: Lactate or Anaerobic Threshold; L5 - Level 5: Sub-Maximum to Maximum Effort

Endurance Program

50 minutes to 5 Hours
30 Minutes per Day

PROGRAM GUIDELINES

Who

This program is for those who bike on average 3–5 days per week and whose cycling sessions vary in length, but generally last between 45 minutes and 4 hours (sometimes more). You have been a consistent cyclist for at least several months or have a specific amount of time to devote to your fitness program and want to ensure you get in a challenging week of training. You may or may not have experience with organized cycling events but would like to take your training to the next level. You have your eyes set on a riding a century ride.

What and How

This program is your map for each week of bike training. Your week incorporates: recovery, several high intensity options (intervals, tempo), hill training and long/long fartlek training sessions. This program comes with multiple options within each session category. You can change sessions each week as you wish, mixing them up to keep your training fun and challenging. Sessions are listed within each category with increasing difficulty. I recommend starting at the top of the list and making your way down as your fitness increases.

If you have been cycling 3–4 days per week, I recommend you continue doing so for a few weeks before you increase the quantity of sessions per week. If you have been cycling 4 or more sessions per week, continue to do so while adding 1–2 sessions after several weeks. Take additional recovery sessions or rest days, as needed.

Rules

• Use the guidelines in your program to plug in training sessions on given days.

• Do not do high intensity options (intervals, tempo), hill sessions on back-to-back days. Take a recovery day between each of these sessions.

- Do each workout at the prescribed training level. For example, do your recovery sessions at L1–L2, which is a very easy effort. This will help you get the most out of your more challenging workouts and allow for your best overall training effect.

- After 2–3 weeks of executing this program, do one active recovery week in which you decrease the overall time and intensity of each session by 20–30%. The following week you can jump back up to a full week. Repeat this pattern with 2–3 weeks, followed by an easier week. This is a means to periodize your program and is necessary to get the full effect from your training.

Strength Training

If you have done consistent strength training prior to going into this program and you have the time available, continue to execute your strength training routine while adding in the strength and core exercises shown in this program. If you have not been doing any strength work, execute the strength and core exercises as designated in this program, while using the above rules as a guide.

ENDURANCE PROGRAM: 50 MINUTES TO 5 HOURS 30 MINUTES PER DAY

Day 1

STRETCH :15

REST DAY

Day 2

STRETCH :15

BIKE SESSION: Choose one workout from one of these lists: INTERVALS or TEMPO

Walking Lunges: 3x15

Side Shuffle Lunges: 3x15

Push-ups: 3x15 (full plank or knees-down push-ups, whichever you can do while maintaining a straight torso)

Ab crunches: 70

Day 3: RECOVERY

STRETCH :15

REST DAY, CROSS-TRAIN, or BIKE :50 (L1–L2)

Day 4

STRETCH :15

BIKE SESSION*: Choose one workout from this list: HILLS.

Walking Lunges: 3x15

Side Shuffle Lunges: 3x15

Push-ups: 3x15 (full plank or knees-down push-ups, whichever you can do while maintaining a straight torso)

Ab crunches: 70

*If you are still feeling tired from your Day 2 Session, do Day 5 RECOVERY workout today and do your HILLS session on Day 5.

Day 5: RECOVERY

STRETCH :15

REST DAY, CROSS-TRAIN, or BIKE :50 (L1–L2)

Day 6

STRETCH :15

BIKE 1:10 (L1–L3)

Day 7

STRETCH :15

BIKE SESSION: Choose one workout from the LONG or LONG/FARTLEK session list. Start with the distance you are currently doing with your long ride, then gradually work your way down the list each week. After 2–3 weeks of executing your long ride on this day, do one active recovery week in which you decrease the overall time and intensity of this session by 20–30%.

Day 2 SESSION

Choose *one* workout from *one* of the below session categories.

INTERVALS:
50 minutes to 1 hour
10 minutes

Choose a flat route for this workout.

DAY 2 INTERVALS

INTERVAL 1
BIKE :50 (L1–L4)

Warm up at L1–L2 for :10

4x30 second pick-ups with 1 minute at L2 between each

1, 2, 3, 2, 1 minute at L3–L4 with 2 minutes at L2 between each

4x30 second pick-ups with 1 minute at L2 between each

Cool down the remaining time at L1–L2

L1 - Level 1: Recovery; **L2** - Level 2: Aerobic; **L3** - Level 3: High-End Aerobic to Low Anaerobic; **L4** - Level 4: Lactate or Anaerobic Threshold; **L5** - Level 5: Sub-Maximum to Maximum Effort

INTERVAL 2
BIKE :50 (L1–L4)

Warm up at L1–L2 for :10

2x30 second pick-ups with 1 minute at L2 between each

6x2 minutes at L4 with 1:30 minutes at L2 between each

2x1 minute at L4 with 1 minute at L2 between each

2x30 second pick-ups with 1 minute at L2 between each

Cool down the remaining time at L1–L2

L1 - Level 1: Recovery; L2 - Level 2: Aerobic; L3 - Level 3: High-End Aerobic to Low Anaerobic;
L4 - Level 4: Lactate or Anaerobic Threshold; L5 - Level 5: Sub-Maximum to Maximum Effort

DAY 2 INTERVALS

INTERVAL 3
BIKE 1:00 (L1–L4)

Warm up at L1–L2 for :10

4x30 second pick-ups with 1 minute at L2 between each

2x2 minutes at L4 with 1:30 minutes at L2 between each

2x4 minutes at L3 with 3 minutes at L2 between each

2x3 minutes at L4 with 2 minutes at L2 between each

Cool down the remaining time at L1–L2

L1 - Level 1: Recovery; L2 - Level 2: Aerobic; L3 - Level 3: High-End Aerobic to Low Anaerobic; L4 - Level 4: Lactate or Anaerobic Threshold; L5 - Level 5: Sub-Maximum to Maximum Effort

INTERVAL 4
BIKE 1:00 (L1–L4)

Warm up at L1–L2 for :10

4x1 minute pick-ups with 30 seconds at L2 between each

2, 3, 4, 3, 2 minutes at L4. Take the same amount of at L2 between each as the interval prior.

Cool down the remaining time at L1–L2

L1 - Level 1: Recovery; L2 - Level 2: Aerobic; L3 - Level 3: High-End Aerobic to Low Anaerobic; L4 - Level 4: Lactate or Anaerobic Threshold; L5 - Level 5: Sub-Maximum to Maximum Effort

DAY 2 INTERVALS

INTERVAL 5
BIKE 1:10 (L1–L4)

Warm up at L1–L2 for :15

4x1 minute pick-ups with 30 seconds at L2 between each

5x4 minutes at L3–L4 with 3 minutes at L2 between each

Cool down the remaining time at L1–L2

L1 - Level 1: Recovery; **L2** - Level 2: Aerobic; **L3** - Level 3: High-End Aerobic to Low Anaerobic; **L4** - Level 4: Lactate or Anaerobic Threshold; **L5** - Level 5: Sub-Maximum to Maximum Effort

INTERVAL 6
BIKE 1:10 (L1–L4)

Warm up at L1–L2 for :15

4x1 minute pick-ups with 30 seconds at L2 between each

1, 2, 3, 4, 4, 3, 2, 1 minute at L4. Ride at L2 between each for the same amount of time as the interval prior.

Cool down the remaining time at L1–L2

L1 - Level 1: Recovery; L2 - Level 2: Aerobic; L3 - Level 3: High-End Aerobic to Low Anaerobic;
L4 - Level 4: Lactate or Anaerobic Threshold; L5 - Level 5: Sub-Maximum to Maximum Effort

TEMPO:
50 minutes to 1 hour 10 minutes

These sessions can be done anywhere and on any type of terrain. Tempo rides include a designated period of time in which you ride at a specific and consistent pace. The goal is to ride the designated tempo time, sustaining the allotted pace.

TEMPO 1
BIKE :50 (L1–L4)

Warm up at L1–L2 for :10

8 minutes at L3
2 minutes at L2
8 minutes at L3
4 minutes at L4

Cool down the remaining time at L1–L2

L1 - Level 1: Recovery; L2 - Level 2: Aerobic; L3 - Level 3: High-End Aerobic to Low Anaerobic;
L4 - Level 4: Lactate or Anaerobic Threshold; L5 - Level 5: Sub-Maximum to Maximum Effort

TEMPO 2
BIKE :50 (L1–L4)

DAY 2 TEMPO

Warm up at L1–L2 for :15

12 minutes at L3
2 minutes at L2
6 minutes at L3–L4

Cool down the remaining time at L1–L2

L1 - Level 1: Recovery; L2 - Level 2: Aerobic; L3 - Level 3: High-End Aerobic to Low Anaerobic; L4 - Level 4: Lactate or Anaerobic Threshold; L5 - Level 5: Sub-Maximum to Maximum Effort

DAY 2 TEMPO

TEMPO 3
BIKE 1:00 (L1–L4)

Warm up at L1–L2 for :15

15 minutes at L3
5 minutes at L4

Cool down the remaining time at L1– L2

L1 - Level 1: Recovery; L2 - Level 2: Aerobic; L3 - Level 3: High-End Aerobic to Low Anaerobic; L4 - Level 4: Lactate or Anaerobic Threshold; L5 - Level 5: Sub-Maximum to Maximum Effort

TEMPO 4
BIKE 1:00 (L1–L4)

Warm up at L1–L2 for :15

14 minutes at L3
2 minutes at L2
6 minutes at L4

**Cool down the remaining time at L1–
L2**

L1 - Level 1: Recovery; L2 - Level 2: Aerobic; L3 - Level 3: High-End Aerobic to Low Anaerobic;
L4 - Level 4: Lactate or Anaerobic Threshold; L5 - Level 5: Sub-Maximum to Maximum Effort

DAY 2 TEMPO

TEMPO 5
BIKE 1:10 (L1–L4)

Warm up at L1–L2 for :20

12 minutes at L3
10 minutes at L3–L4

Cool down the remaining time at L1–L2

L1 - Level 1: Recovery; L2 - Level 2: Aerobic; L3 - Level 3: High-End Aerobic to Low Anaerobic; L4 - Level 4: Lactate or Anaerobic Threshold; L5 - Level 5: Sub-Maximum to Maximum Effort

TEMPO 6
<u>BIKE 1:10 (L1–L4)</u>

Warm up at L1–L2 for :20

14 minutes at L3

3 minutes at L2

8 minutes at L4

Cool down the remaining time at L1–L2

L1 - Level 1: Recovery; **L2** - Level 2: Aerobic; **L3** - Level 3: High-End Aerobic to Low Anaerobic; **L4** - Level 4: Lactate or Anaerobic Threshold; **L5** - Level 5: Sub-Maximum to Maximum Effort

Day 4 SESSION

Choose *one* workout from *one* of the
below session categories.

HILLS:
50 minutes to 1 hour
10 minutes

Hill workouts include: increasing pace on hills within a ride, hill repeats, and sustained hill efforts. If you have more time for this workout and you have been consistently doing hill training prior to taking on this program, add 1–2 more hill efforts within the workout.

DAY 4 HILLS

HILLS 1
<u>BIKE :50 (L1–L4)</u>

Choose a hilly BIKE route that includes at least 6–8 hills that take 1 minute or less to ride up

Warm up at L1–L2 for :10 on flatter terrain prior to arriving at your first hill effort

When you come to a hill ride it at L3–L4. Continue your ride to the next hill at L2, then repeat the L3–L4 effort on the next hill.

Once 6-8 hills are completed cool down the remaining time at L1–L2

L1 - Level 1: Recovery; **L2** - Level 2: Aerobic; **L3** - Level 3: High-End Aerobic to Low Anaerobic;
L4 - Level 4: Lactate or Anaerobic Threshold; **L5** - Level 5: Sub-Maximum to Maximum Effort

HILLS 2
BIKE :50 (L1–L4)

Warm up at L1–L2 for :10 on flat terrain

Choose a hill that takes you 45 seconds to 1 minute to ride up

BIKE this hill 8x at L4. Between each, coast slowly to the bottom, take an additional 20 seconds recovery before executing your next hill.

Cool down the remaining time at L1–L2

L1 - Level 1: Recovery; **L2** - Level 2: Aerobic; **L3** - Level 3: High-End Aerobic to Low Anaerobic; **L4** - Level 4: Lactate or Anaerobic Threshold; **L5** - Level 5: Sub-Maximum to Maximum Effort

DAY 4 HILLS

HILLS 3
BIKE 1:00 (L1–L4)

Warm up at L1–L2 for :15 on flat terrain

Choose a hill that takes you 1:30 minutes to ride up

BIKE this hill 8x at L3–L4. Coast slowly to the bottom of the hill and immediately execute your next hill.

Cool down the remaining time at L1–L2

L1 - Level 1: Recovery; L2 - Level 2: Aerobic; L3 - Level 3: High-End Aerobic to Low Anaerobic; L4 - Level 4: Lactate or Anaerobic Threshold; L5 - Level 5: Sub-Maximum to Maximum Effort

HILLS 4
BIKE 1:00 (L1–L4)

DAY 4 HILLS

Warm up at L1–L2 for :15 on flat
    terrain

Choose a hill that takes you 1:30
    minutes to ride up

BIKE this hill 8x at L4, extending
    your effort for an additional 15
    seconds over the top and as the
    terrain flattens out. Coast slowly
    to the bottom of the hill and
    immediately execute your next
    hill-extension.

Cool down the remaining time at L1–
    L2

L1 - Level 1: Recovery; L2 - Level 2: Aerobic; L3 - Level 3: High-End Aerobic to Low Anaerobic;
L4 - Level 4: Lactate or Anaerobic Threshold; L5 - Level 5: Sub-Maximum to Maximum Effort

DAY 4 HILLS

HILLS 5
BIKE 1:10 (L1–L4)

Warm up at L1–L2 for :15 on flat terrain

Choose a long gradual hill that is 1 mile or further in length

Start up the hill riding 1 minute at L4, continue up the hill for 1 minute at L2. Repeat this process 8x as you continue making your way up the hill.

If you cannot maintain an L2 effort during recovery, then extend the recovery interval.

L1 - Level 1: Recovery; **L2** - Level 2: Aerobic; **L3** - Level 3: High-End Aerobic to Low Anaerobic; **L4** - Level 4: Lactate or Anaerobic Threshold; **L5** - Level 5: Sub-Maximum to Maximum Effort

If you reach the top of the hill prior to finishing the set, then turn around and execute recovery on a down slope before riding up again.

Cool down the remaining time at L1–L2

L1 - Level 1: Recovery; L2 - Level 2: Aerobic; L3 - Level 3: High-End Aerobic to Low Anaerobic;
L4 - Level 4: Lactate or Anaerobic Threshold; L5 - Level 5: Sub-Maximum to Maximum Effort

DAY 4 HILLS

HILLS 6
BIKE 1:10 (L1–L4)

Warm up at L1–L2 for :15 on flat terrain

Choose a hill that takes you 1:30–2 minutes to ride up

BIKE this hill 8x at L4, extending your effort for an additional 20 seconds over the top and as the terrain flattens out. Coast slowly to the bottom of the hill and immediately execute your next hill-extension.

Cool down the remaining time at L1–L2

L1 - Level 1: Recovery; L2 - Level 2: Aerobic; L3 - Level 3: High-End Aerobic to Low Anaerobic; L4 - Level 4: Lactate or Anaerobic Threshold; L5 - Level 5: Sub-Maximum to Maximum Effort

Day 7 SESSION

Choose *one* workout below.

LONG OR LONG/FARTLEK: 3 hours 30 minutes to 5 hours 30 minutes

The LONG BIKE is your longest ride of the week. Fartlek, or speed-play, is typically a whimsical and spontaneous speed session—you increase your pace when and how much you wish, as you go. Use the guidelines to approximate your efforts within each LONG/FARTLEK session. You do not have to execute the speed increases in the order they are listed. You can add them in as you wish.

DAY 7 LONG/FARTLEK

LONG/FARTLEK 1
BIKE 3:30

Warm up at L1–L2 for :30

Within the rest of the ride do the following when you wish:

8 speed increases for: 1 minute between telephone poles or trees, or a similar length/ distance. Take a similar length of time/distance at L2 between each.

BIKE the remaining time at L2–L3

L1 - Level 1: Recovery; L2 - Level 2: Aerobic; L3 - Level 3: High-End Aerobic to Low Anaerobic; L4 - Level 4: Lactate or Anaerobic Threshold; L5 - Level 5: Sub-Maximum to Maximum Effort

LONG/FARTLEK 2
BIKE 3:30

Warm up at L1–L2 for :30

Within the rest of the ride do the following when you wish:

4 speed increases for: 1 minute between telephone poles or trees, or a similar length/distance. Take a similar length of time/distance at L2 between each.

3 speed increases for: 2 minutes or a half mile in length. Use your watch or an object en route as a finish point.

2 speed increase for: 3 minutes or a mile in length. Use your watch or an object en route as a finish point.

L1 - Level 1: Recovery; **L2** - Level 2: Aerobic; **L3** - Level 3: High-End Aerobic to Low Anaerobic; **L4** - Level 4: Lactate or Anaerobic Threshold; **L5** - Level 5: Sub-Maximum to Maximum Effort

DAY 7 LONG/FARTLEK

DAY 7 LONG/FARTLEK

Take as much time as you wish at L2 between each.

BIKE the remaining time at L2–L3

L1 - Level 1: Recovery; L2 - Level 2: Aerobic; L3 - Level 3: High-End Aerobic to Low Anaerobic;
L4 - Level 4: Lactate or Anaerobic Threshold; L5 - Level 5: Sub-Maximum to Maximum Effort

LONG 3
BIKE 3:45 (L1–L4)

Warm up at L1–L2 for :45

BIKE L2–L3 for :25
BIKE L3–L4 for :05
BIKE L4 for :15

BIKE the remaining time at L2–L3

DAY 7 LONG/FARTLEK

L1 - Level 1: Recovery; **L2** - Level 2: Aerobic; **L3** - Level 3: High-End Aerobic to Low Anaerobic; **L4** - Level 4: Lactate or Anaerobic Threshold; **L5** - Level 5: Sub-Maximum to Maximum Effort

DAY 7 LONG/FARTLEK

LONG 4
BIKE 3:45 (L1–L4)

Warm up at L1–L2 for :45

BIKE L3 for :15
BIKE L4 for :05
BIKE L3 for :15
BIKE L4 for :05

BIKE the remaining time at L2–L3

LONG/FARTLEK 5
<u>BIKE 4:00</u>

Warm up at L1–L2 for :45

Within the rest of the ride do the following when you wish:

13 speed increases, each less than 1 minute or approximately a half mile. Use your watch or an object en route as a finish point.

Take as much time as you wish at L2 between each.

BIKE the remaining time at L2–L3

DAY 7 LONG/FARTLEK

L1 - Level 1: Recovery; **L2** - Level 2: Aerobic; **L3** - Level 3: High-End Aerobic to Low Anaerobic;
L4 - Level 4: Lactate or Anaerobic Threshold; **L5** - Level 5: Sub-Maximum to Maximum Effort

DAY 7 LONG/FARTLEK

LONG/FARTLEK 6
BIKE 4:00

Warm up at L1–L2 for :45

Within the rest of the ride do the following when you wish:

8 speed increases for: 30 seconds between telephone poles or trees, or a similar length/ distance. Take a similar length of time/distance at L2 between each.

4 speed increases for: 4 minutes or approximately a mile. Use your watch or an object en route as a finish point.

Take as much time as you wish at L2 between each.

BIKE the remaining time at L2–L3

L1 - Level 1: Recovery; L2 - Level 2: Aerobic; L3 - Level 3: High-End Aerobic to Low Anaerobic;
L4 - Level 4: Lactate or Anaerobic Threshold; L5 - Level 5: Sub-Maximum to Maximum Effort

LONG 7
BIKE 4:15 (L1–L4)

Warm up at L1–L2 for :50

BIKE L2–L3 for :25
BIKE L1–L2 for :20
BIKE L2–L3 for :15
BIKE L4 for :05

BIKE the remaining time at L2–L3

DAY 7 LONG/FARTLEK

L1 - Level 1: Recovery; L2 - Level 2: Aerobic; L3 - Level 3: High-End Aerobic to Low Anaerobic;
L4 - Level 4: Lactate or Anaerobic Threshold; L5 - Level 5: Sub-Maximum to Maximum Effort

LONG 8
BIKE 4:15 (L1–L4)

Warm up at L1–L2 for :45

BIKE L2–L3 for :25
BIKE L1–L2 for :20
BIKE L2–L3 for :15
BIKE L3–L4 for :10
BIKE L4 for :05

BIKE the remaining time at L2–L3

L1 - Level 1: Recovery; L2 - Level 2: Aerobic; L3 - Level 3: High-End Aerobic to Low Anaerobic; L4 - Level 4: Lactate or Anaerobic Threshold; L5 - Level 5: Sub-Maximum to Maximum Effort

LONG/FARTLEK 9
BIKE 4:30

Warm up at L1–L2 for :50

Within the rest of the ride do the following when you wish:

14 speed increases for: 1 minute between telephone poles or trees, or a similar length/ distance. Take a similar length of time/distance at L2 between each.

BIKE the remaining time at L2–L3

DAY 7 LONG/FARTLEK

L1 - Level 1: Recovery; L2 - Level 2: Aerobic; L3 - Level 3: High-End Aerobic to Low Anaerobic;
L4 - Level 4: Lactate or Anaerobic Threshold; L5 - Level 5: Sub-Maximum to Maximum Effort

DAY 7 LONG/FARTLEK

LONG/FARTLEK 10
BIKE 4:45

Warm up at L1–L2 for :50

Within the rest of the ride do the following when you wish:

6 speed increases for: 1 minute, between telephone poles or trees, or a similar length/distance. Take a similar length of time/distance at L2 between each.

4 speed increases for: 2 minutes or a half mile in length. Use your watch or an object en route as a finish point.

3 speed increase for: 3 minutes or a mile in length. Use your watch or an object en route as a finish point.

L1 - Level 1: Recovery; L2 - Level 2: Aerobic; L3 - Level 3: High-End Aerobic to Low Anaerobic; L4 - Level 4: Lactate or Anaerobic Threshold; L5 - Level 5: Sub-Maximum to Maximum Effort

Take as much time as you wish at L2 between each.

BIKE the remaining time at L2–L3

DAY 7 LONG/FARTLEK

L1 - Level 1: Recovery; L2 - Level 2: Aerobic; L3 - Level 3: High-End Aerobic to Low Anaerobic;
L4 - Level 4: Lactate or Anaerobic Threshold; L5 - Level 5: Sub-Maximum to Maximum Effort

DAY 7 LONG/FARTLEK

LONG 11
BIKE 5:00 (L1–L4)

Warm up at L1–L2 for :45

BIKE L2–L3 for :25
BIKE L3–L4 for :05
BIKE L4 for :05
BIKE L3–L4 for :05
BIKE L4 for :05

BIKE the remaining time at L2–L3

L1 - Level 1: Recovery; **L2** - Level 2: Aerobic; **L3** - Level 3: High-End Aerobic to Low Anaerobic; **L4** - Level 4: Lactate or Anaerobic Threshold; **L5** - Level 5: Sub-Maximum to Maximum Effort

LONG 12
BIKE 5:00 (L1–L4)

Warm up at L1–L2 for :45

BIKE L3 for :15
BIKE L4 for :05
BIKE L3 for :15
BIKE L4 for :05

BIKE the remaining time at L2–L3

L1 - Level 1: Recovery; L2 - Level 2: Aerobic; L3 - Level 3: High-End Aerobic to Low Anaerobic;
L4 - Level 4: Lactate or Anaerobic Threshold; L5 - Level 5: Sub-Maximum to Maximum Effort

LONG/FARTLEK 13
BIKE 5:15

Warm up at L1–L2 for :45

Within the rest of the ride do the following when you wish:

18 speed increases, each less than 1 minute or approximately a half mile. Use your watch or an object en route as a finish point.

Take as much time as you wish between each

BIKE the remaining time at L2–L3

L1 - Level 1: Recovery; **L2** - Level 2: Aerobic; **L3** - Level 3: High-End Aerobic to Low Anaerobic;
L4 - Level 4: Lactate or Anaerobic Threshold; **L5** - Level 5: Sub-Maximum to Maximum Effort

LONG/FARTLEK 14
BIKE 5:15

Warm up at L1–L2 for :45

Within the rest of the ride do the following when you wish:

8 speed increases for: 30 seconds between telephone poles or trees, or a similar length/distance. Take a similar length of time/distance at L2 between each.

5 speed increases for: 4 minutes or approximately a mile. Use your watch or an object en route as a finish point.

Take as much time as you wish at L2 between each.

BIKE the remaining time at L2–L3

L1 - Level 1: Recovery; L2 - Level 2: Aerobic; L3 - Level 3: High-End Aerobic to Low Anaerobic; L4 - Level 4: Lactate or Anaerobic Threshold; L5 - Level 5: Sub-Maximum to Maximum Effort

DAY 7 LONG/FARTLEK

DAY 7 LONG/FARTLEK

LONG 15
BIKE 5:30 (L1–L4)

Warm up at L1–L2 for :45

BIKE L2–L3 for :25
BIKE L1–L2 for :20
BIKE L2–L3 for :15
BIKE L4 for :05
BIKE L2–L3 for :15
BIKE L4 for :05

BIKE the remaining time at L2–L3

L1 - Level 1: Recovery; **L2** - Level 2: Aerobic; **L3** - Level 3: High-End Aerobic to Low Anaerobic;
L4 - Level 4: Lactate or Anaerobic Threshold; **L5** - Level 5: Sub-Maximum to Maximum Effort

LONG 16
BIKE 5:30 (L1–L4)

Warm up at L1–L2 for :45

BIKE L2–L3 for :25
BIKE L1–L2 for :20
BIKE L2–L3 for :15
BIKE L3–L4 for :10
BIKE L2–L3 for :15
BIKE L3–L4 for :10

BIKE the remaining time at L2–L3

L1 - Level 1: Recovery; **L2** - Level 2: Aerobic; **L3** - Level 3: High-End Aerobic to Low Anaerobic; **L4** - Level 4: Lactate or Anaerobic Threshold; **L5** - Level 5: Sub-Maximum to Maximum Effort

ABOUT THE AUTHOR

Terri Schneider is an ultra-endurance athlete, writer, speaker, coach and sport psychology consultant. She has authored *Dirty Inspirations: Lessons from the Trenches of Extreme Endurance Sports* and *Triathlon Revolution: Training, Technique and Inspiration*, co-authored *Triathlete's Guide to Mental Training*, and contributed to several other books. As a former 10-year professional triathlete focusing on the IRONMAN® distance, she then segued 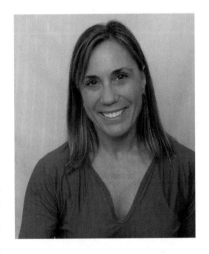 into adventure racing with the inception of the Eco Challenge in 1995, as well as ultrarunning and mountaineering. Terri earned a bachelor's degree in exercise physiology as well as a master's degree in sport psychology with a research emphasis on risk taking and team dynamics.

Her writing contributions, profile, and interviews have been featured in over 100 publications and websites around the world including *Time, Psychology Today, Rolling Stone, Runner's World, Triathlete, Cosmopolitan, Glamour, Outside, Oxygen, USA Today,* and *The New York Times*.

While Santa Cruz, CA remains her home base, she spends time each year volunteering in Bhutan while continuing to explore and adventure around the globe, sharing her experiences through her speaking, writing and photography. For more info go to www.terrischneider.net.

TAKE IT TO THE NEXT LEVEL WITH THESE
MUST-HAVE WORKOUT PROGRAMS

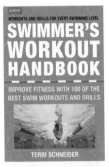

Swimmer's Workout Handbook

978-1-57826-682-1
E-Book: 978-1-57826-683-8
Improve fitness with 100 of the best swim workouts and drills.

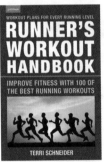

Runner's Workout Handbook

978-1-57826-697-5
E-Book: 978-1-57826-698-2
Perfect fit for both recreational and fitness runners, as well as competitive athletes.

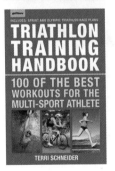

Triathlon Training Handbook

978-1-57826-724-8
E-Book: 978-1-57826-725-5
A complete guide to innovative, full-spectrum fitness planning for triathletes, or those interested in a cross-training fitness program.

Available where books are sold
Also available at www.getfitnow.com

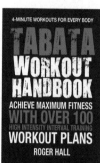

Tabata Workout Handbook

978-1-57826-561-9
E-Book: 978-1-57826-562-6
The original collection of HIIT workouts perfect for all fitness levels.

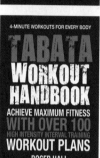

Tabata Workout Handbook Volume 2

978-1-57826-722-4
E-Book: 978-1-57826-723-1
Take your tabata to the next level with 100 new HIIT workouts, including barbell and dumbbell tabatas.

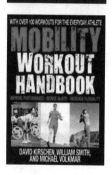

The Mobility Workout Handbook

978-1-57826-619-7
E-Book: 978-1-57826-620-3
Improve fitness and reduce injury with more than 100 mobility workouts.

Available where books are sold
Also available at www.getfitnow.com